## DO YOU KNOW . . .

- The number of days of bed rest now considered optimal after a back injury
- Alternating hot and cold showers can effectively relieve chronic backache
- An herb called devil's claw is a heavenly remedy for the pain, inflammation, and headache that accompany arthritis and spondylosis
- Elderberry wine can relieve sciatica
- The teaspoon of sugar you put in your coffee may be hurting your back
- In craniosacral therapy, light pressure is applied *to your head,* which in turn helps heal an ailing back

PLUS NATURAL ALTERNATIVES TO TREAT
SPRAINED BACK, SLIPPED DISK, DEGENERATIVE
DISK DISEASE, ARTHRITIS, SPONDYLOLYSIS AND
SPONDYLOLISTHESIS, ANKYLOSING
SPONDYLITIS, SCOLIOSIS, SPINAL STENOSIS,
FIBROMYALGIA, OSTEOPOROSIS AND
OSTEOMALACIA, AND FRACTURES

**THE DELL NATURAL MEDICINE LIBRARY**

PREVENTION, HEALING, SYMPTOM RELIEF . . .
FROM NATURE TO YOU

Also available from the Dell Natural Medicine Library:

NATURAL MEDICINE FOR HEART DISEASE

NATURAL MEDICINE FOR BREAST CANCER

NATURAL MEDICINE FOR ARTHRITIS

NATURAL MEDICINE FOR DIABETES

# THE DELL
# NATURAL MEDICINE LIBRARY

# NATURAL MEDICINE
# FOR
# BACK PAIN

# Deborah Mitchell

*Foreword by Robert M. Giller, M.D.*

A Lynn Sonberg Book

A Dell Book

Published by
Dell Publishing
a division of
Bantam Doubleday Dell Publishing Group, Inc.
1540 Broadway
New York, New York 10036

IMPORTANT NOTE: Neither this nor any other book should be used as a substitute for professional medical care or treatment. It is advisable to seek the guidance of a physician or other qualified health practitioner before implementing any of the approaches to health suggested in this book. This book was written to provide selected information to the public concerning conventional and alternative medical treatments for back pain. Research in this field is ongoing and subject to interpretation. Although we have made all reasonable efforts to include the most up-to-date and accurate information in this book, there is no guarantee that what we know about this complex subject won't change with time. The reader should bear in mind that this book is not intended to take the place of medical advice from a trained medical professional. Readers are advised to consult a physician or other qualified health professional regarding treatment of all of their health problems. Neither the publisher, the producer, nor the authors take any responsibility for any possible consequences from any treatment, action, or application of medicine or preparation by any person reading or following the information in this book.

ISBN: 0-440-22171-4

Published by arrangement with:
Lynn Sonberg Book Associates
10 West 86 Street
New York, NY 10024

Printed in the United States of America
Published simultaneously in Canada

May 1997

10  9  8  7  6  5  4  3  2  1

OPM

# ACKNOWLEDGMENTS

The author gratefully acknowledges the assistance provided by Robert M. Giller, M.D., and thanks him for his expeditious and thoughtful review. She also thanks the nameless backache sufferers who shared their experiences with her. Two others deserve special mention: Lynn Sonberg, for her guidance; and Tim Schaefer, the author's ever-patient husband.

# CONTENTS

## PART III   MEDICAL THERAPIES FOR BACK
PAIN

# FOREWORD

You have in your hands a book I have personally subtitled "Everything You Want to Know About Back Pain But Your Doctor Could Not Tell You." If you have tried conventional back-pain treatments and had little or no success; if you are looking for safe, natural ways to prevent, control, and/or eliminate chronic or acute back pain, *Natural Medicine for Back Pain,* a comprehensive, self-help primer, is for you. Utilizing an easy-to-read, well-organized format, it presents answers to questions such as What is back pain? What causes it? What is the role of the mind in pain? and most important, What can I do to reduce/eliminate/prevent back pain?

The majority of this book answers this last question by offering a smorgasbord of natural therapies, as well as some conventional ones, that allow you to take control of your back pain. Results of the latest studies show that the best treatment for most people who suffer with back pain is PET: patience, exercise, and time. When holistic therapies are added to this prescription, such as those explained in Part II of this book, you can gently and safely speed up the healing process. You will learn how to choose the best therapies for you. Each therapeutic option in this book is explored from several angles: how to treat yourself or, if need be, how to find an appropriate practitioner; what to expect from various therapists and practitioners; and what kind of results you can achieve. These holistic treatments can be tried without fear of adverse effects. In fact they often provide people with many more benefits than just back-pain relief. What are those benefits? Part II reveals those as well.

Whether you choose to complement your conventional treatment with one or more natural approaches or to explore the natural route exclusively, always see your physician first for a complete medical examination to rule out the remote possibility of a serious medical condition. Either way I believe *Natural Medicine for Back Pain* is a reliable resource for you and for everyone with back pain who wants to take control of his or her health and well-being.

ROBERT M. GILLER, M.D.
AUTHOR, *Natural Prescriptions*

# Introduction

The fact that you're reading this book probably means you're among the estimated 80 percent or more of people who now have, once had, or will again experience, back pain. Perhaps you've just experienced the often crippling— but fortunately usually transient—pain of an acute attack. Maybe you are nursing your back after such an incident, or maybe you have chronic back pain. You may have tried bed rest and are taking it easy. Perhaps you've visited your doctor and are taking pain medication. Chances are good you are among the 80 to 90 percent of patients who improve within two months with or without medical intervention. But you would like relief *now*. And you also would like to know how you can prevent backache from occurring again. Because the fact is back pain is rarely a onetime event. Once you have had a back injury—a pulled muscle, sprain, strain, or something more serious—you are four times more likely to experience repeat pain. Approximately 60 percent of people who have acute, debilitating low back pain have a repeat attack within two years.

If you are tired of suffering with back pain and are ready

to try a natural approach to healing, this book will introduce you to holistic therapies to keep your back, your body, and your mind healthy so that you can reduce, prevent, or eliminate the occurrence or risk of backache.

*Natural Medicine for Back Pain* is not intended to take the place of advice and information from medical and health care professionals. Natural medicine does not replace conventional biomedicine; rather, often it is complementary to conventional medical approaches and serves to broaden the therapeutic possibilities. Conventional medicine treats symptoms, and the focus is on the ailment; natural medicine treats the entire person, with consideration, in most cases, of the body, mind, and spirit.

Within these pages you may find concepts you have never thought about or experienced before. Natural medicine has been likened to opening windows to one's body, mind, and soul. It exposes you to new insights and information about yourself, the intricate interrelationships among the systems in your body, and the special relationship between body and mind. This book doesn't claim to have all the solutions. Its purpose is to expand your options, introduce you to new possibilities for back-pain relief, and help you become better acquainted with your best friend—your body—and show you how you can better control your back pain. You should always, however, check with your primary-care physician before using the natural therapies described in this book. This is especially crucial if you are pregnant or are being treated for any ongoing medical condition.

In chapters 1 through 3 you will become familiar with your back and its relationship to the rest of your body as we look at "back basics" and some guidelines to daily care. In Chapter 4 "The Mind-Body Connection" you will get answers to questions such as What effect do my emotions and feelings have on back pain? and How can I use my mind to control my pain?

In Part II you are presented with a comprehensive chart that allows you to locate quickly either the treatment, prevention, and maintenance, or the pain-control approach you want to take for acute or chronic back pain. How can applying pressure to a spot on my foot relieve back pain? and Which herbs can I use to relieve the stress and tension that are contributing to my back pain? are just two of the many questions answered in Part II. Part III discusses some of the medical therapies for back pain. A wealth of information to help you locate products, organizations, further reading materials, and other resources concerning back pain is given at the end of this book.

We hope this volume helps you lead a more active, joyful, and healthy life, one that is free of the pain and challenges of backache.

# PART I

# YOU AND YOUR BACK PAIN

# CHAPTER ONE

# Understanding Back Pain

We are a nation of people with back pain. At any point in time 16 percent of adults between the ages of twenty-five and seventy-four are experiencing low back pain, defined by the National Health and Nutritional Examination Survey II (NHNESII) as an episode lasting two weeks or longer. Approximately 1 percent of Americans are chronically disabled with back pain and another 1 percent are temporarily disabled. Among the most common afflictions that affect Americans, back pain is second only to the common cold. The good news is most back pain can be prevented, reduced significantly, or eliminated naturally, without drugs or surgery, and without lying in bed staring at the ceiling for days or weeks on end.

It is estimated that Americans spend more than $16 billion a year for various back-pain treatments. That's a lot of painkillers and doctor visits, as well as a lot of time lost from work, school, and play. Before we can change how you treat and manage back pain, we need to become familiar with what pain is and with some "back basics."

## Categories and Types of Back Pain

Pain can be categorized broadly as either acute or chronic. Because pain is a very personal experience and a difficult thing to quantify and describe objectively, these terms are used loosely when referring to any type of pain. Generally acute back pain is one way the body responds to a physically or emotionally stressful situation, such as infection, muscle strain, inflammation, or anger, that resolves within a reasonable amount of time, depending on the extent of the original injury. Researchers have determined that 80 to 90 percent of patients improve within approximately two months, even without medical intervention.

Chronic pain is a more complex issue, involving continuous pain past a reasonable time for healing to occur and complicated by other factors, such as economic, social, and psychological issues. Sharon, a thirty-eight-year-old teacher, knows about these factors very well. For the past three years she has suffered from chronic low back pain. On most mornings she can function well as long as she takes some pain medication. Occasionally, however, she cannot get out of bed and must call in sick to work. Both her husband and her son are avid skiers and also enjoy hiking and rafting, all sports Sharon had to give up because of her back pain. Like Sharon, many people with chronic pain become depressed about their inability to do all they used to do when they were pain-free. People's emotional state can have a significant impact on their pain, and we discuss this in more depth in Chapter 4.

Another aspect of back pain, acute or chronic, is that the degree of pain is not always an indicator of its clinical seriousness. A simple stretched back muscle may send a brawny man to his knees while a herniated disk may cause a mild backache for weeks or months until it reaches a point when it presses against a nerve and numbs an arm or leg.

## Lumbar, Thoracic, and Cervical Back Pain

There are three main types of back pain, and these correspond to three of the five sections of the spine (see Figure I-1): lumbar (lower back, consisting of five vertebrae), thoracic (middle back, twelve vertebrae), and cervical (neck and upper back, seven vertebrae). The lumbar region is by far the most common site of back pain: Approximately 85 percent of back-pain complaints involve the lower back, compared with 8 percent for the middle back and 7 percent for the upper back. Low back pain comes with a high price tag in terms of money and time. A review of more than six hundred publications that contain data on low back pain indicates that an estimated 2.6 million Americans are permanently disabled because of low back pain. People with low back pain visit health practitioners in droves: In 1990 approximately 16 million visits were made for "sprains, strains, and lumbar disorders," 50 million visits were made to chiropractors, and 2 million visits to physical and occupational therapists.

## Sacrum and Coccyx Pain

Below the lumbar spine is the largest bone in the spine, called the sacrum, which consists of five vertebrae that are fused together. The sacrum bears the concentrated weight of the upper half of the body. As part of the pelvis (the bony structure at the base of the vertebral column), it moves as one unit with it. The sacrum plays a part in a condition called lordosis, or swayback, which is discussed below.

The coccyx, or tailbone, is just below the sacrum and is the fusion of four vertebrae. Although this part of the spine does not help support the body, it serves as a connection point for the gluteus maximus, or the buttocks muscles, and

**I-1 The spinal column**

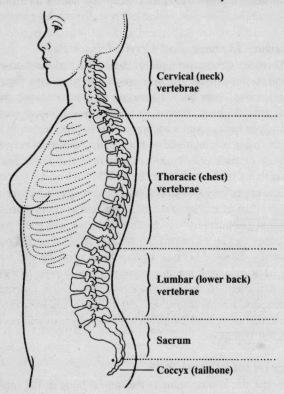

Cervical (neck) vertebrae

Thoracic (chest) vertebrae

Lumbar (lower back) vertebrae

Sacrum

Coccyx (tailbone)

helps to move the legs. Pain in the coccyx is not common, but when it does occur, it is usually associated with a fall, as when someone slips on the ice and the tailbone hits the ground.

## Sciatica

Approximately 25 percent of individuals with back pain also have sciatica, a severe pain felt along the path of the sciatic nerve, which runs along the back of the thigh and down the inside of the leg (see pages 12 and 34 for further information). The pain can affect one or both legs and extends to below the knee, and is usually accompanied by numbness and tingling.

Sciatica is most commonly caused by pressure against the nerve, as when a disk herniates, or from spinal stenosis, which means that the spinal canal is narrow or compromised in some way. We will look at these causes under "Diseases Associated with Back Pain."

## A Lot Goes on Behind Your Back

Just because back pain is common does not mean doctors always know what causes it. Despite the advanced technology of modern medicine, physicians can definitively identify the cause of back pain in only about 15 percent of patients with an acute case. This sounds much worse than it is: Physicians are adept at diagnosing back pain that arises from disease or conditions such as a herniated disk. Yet only 5 to 10 percent of back pain is attributed to such causes. Another small percentage is caused by referred pain associated with vascular, genitourinary, gastrointestinal, and other disorders. But most doctors agree that the vast majority of backaches—about 80 percent—are caused by strained, weak muscles and ligaments, specifically those in the back and abdomen. Strain can occur when you reach for a backhand shot in tennis, step off a curb, pick up your baby, or move a chair. Emotional stress can also cause muscle strain or spasm—a severely contracted, painful muscle.

How can such normal, simple movements cause back pain? To help you understand the answer to this and similar questions, we need to look at (a) the structure of the back—specifically the spine—and see how it functions in relation to the rest of the body; and (b) how other physiological, emotional, environmental, and social factors also affect the back and spine.

## The Holistic Approach to Back Pain

Healthy functioning of the back and spine is intricately linked with many other parts of the body and their condition. If you walk with your toes pointed out to the sides, for example, it causes distortion and stress to the spine. If you are pregnant or have a "beer belly," the excess weight shifts the center of gravity forward and places stress on the lower back. Emotions, diet and nutrition, work and leisure activities, and use of prescription and "recreational" drugs also have an effect on back pain. All of these factors are important reasons to take a holistic, or "whole body," approach to healing your back pain.

## Talking with Your Back

The *spine* is the center of attention of your back. It is composed of vertically arranged spool-shaped bones called *vertebrae* (Figure I-2) which are supported by ligaments and muscles. A healthy spine, viewed from the rear, appears to be straight up and down. From a side view, however, it reveals its true form: an S-shape that is designed to carry body weight and to provide lifting force. The spinal column provides support, stability, and strength, as well as flexibility to the body. If these sound like contrary functions, you're right. This contradiction is one reason why the back is subject to injury: It must be both inflexible (supportive/stabilizing/strong) and flexible on command.

To achieve these seemingly opposite functions, the ligaments and muscles must respond to the positions and circumstances you place yourself in. How they do this is very complex. For our purposes it is sufficient to say that *ligaments* are fibrous tissues that bind bones together and control the motion of the spine. One of these ligaments, the

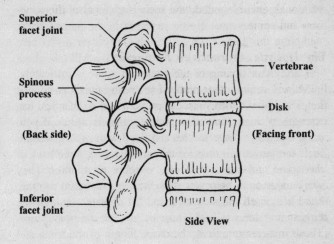

**Superior facet joint**

**Spinous process**

**(Back side)**

**Inferior facet joint**

**Vertebrae**

**Disk**

**(Facing front)**

**Side View**

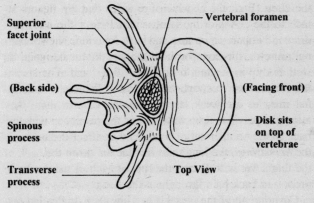

**Superior facet joint**

**(Back side)**

**Spinous process**

**Transverse process**

**Vertebral foramen**

**Disk sits on top of vertebrae**

**(Facing front)**

**Top View**

I-2

yellow ligament, connects the bony back parts of the vertebrae, and is the most elastic structure in the human body. Although this ligament loses its elasticity over time, there are steps you can take to keep it supple. We will talk about this and other ligaments again later.

Muscle strain is the number-one cause of back pain, so it helps to know which muscles are involved so that you can strengthen them. Two main muscle groups are crucial to back function—the extensors and the flexors. The *extensors* include many small muscles that are attached to the back of the spine and cross from one vertebra to another. They work together to help you straighten up, maintain posture, bend backward and sideways, and lift objects. Some of the largest and longest back muscles are the *erector spinae.* These muscles run along the entire length of the spine and are instrumental in moving and supporting the spinal column.

The *flexors* are in the front and include all the abdominal muscles and the hip flexors, which raise the thigh toward the chest. Both the abdominal muscles and hip flexors attach to the pelvis or the lumbar vertebrae and thus have a dramatic impact on posture and back function. The abdominal muscles, for example, help support the lumbar spine as well as help in bending forward, in lifting, and in determining the amount of swayback (lordosis). When the abdominal muscles are weak, as is often the case in men, they allow the pelvis to drop forward and the result can be lower back pain. Another set of muscles that affect the back are the *hamstrings,* the long muscles that run down the back of the thigh. We will discuss the role of each of these muscle groups in back pain throughout the book.

Covering all of the muscles is a fibrous tissue called *fascia.* Some physicians believe this material has a role in back pain, specifically concerning two related conditions known as fibrositis and fibromyalgia. Fibrositis is inflammation of the fibrous tissue that separates the muscles from each other and from other tissues. Fibromyalgia is pain in the fascia and the muscle (see "Fibromyalgia," page 24). Characteristics of these conditions include back pain associated with sleep problems, unresolved emotional issues, and the presence of "trigger points," areas that are very tender and sensitive to the touch. For now the cause of these diseases is unknown, and many doctors question whether they are distinct diseases at all, given that most people improve once they are told their condition is not serious or permanent.

At the back of each vertebra are bony protrusions known as *spinous* and *transverse processes* (Figure I-2). These bones form *neural arches* and collectively make up the spinal canal, which houses and protects the spinal cord. A flat surface called a *facet* is located at the end of each transverse process, and each facet forms a joint with the facets above and below it. The facet joints glide over each other and serve primarily to determine the way the spine moves. Like other joints in the body, the facet joints are susceptible to arthritis, another cause of back pain.

Sandwiched in between each vertebra is a *disk*. Disks play a critical role in the health of the back. Each disk is a collection of ringed fibers and cartilage surrounding a jellylike center, or *nucleus pulposus*. This central portion of disks is composed of 88 percent water, which allows them to act as shock absorbers for the spine. The tough outer fibers of disks, called *annulus fibrosus,* provide the spine with most of its strength. Disks also allow the vertebrae to move, and they distribute weight over the surface of the vertebrae when the spine bends.

Because disks have no blood supply of their own, they depend on a spongelike action to acquire nourishment from nearby tissues so that they can function. During nonweight-bearing rest, such as when you sleep, the disks absorb fluids from surrounding tissues and expand, causing the spine to lengthen as much as one inch. Once you resume weight-bearing activities, the fluid is squeezed back into the adjacent tissues and vertebrae. This cycle of absorption and release of fluids, if allowed to continue without obstruction, helps maintain supple, flexible, healthy disks. When poor posture or loss of flexibility due to poor muscle tone deprives the disks of enough fluids, however, they can become dry, thin, and susceptible to injury. This condition is called *degenerative disk disease,* and later in this book we discuss how you can treat and heal this disease naturally.

Last but not least we have the conveyors of pain, the *nerves.* The superhighway that carries messages between the brain and the rest of the body is the *spinal cord,* which consists of a bundle of nerve cells and fibers that has a diameter the size of your little finger. Along the length of the spinal cord thirty-one pairs of smaller bundles of nerves branch off from between each pair of vertebrae to different parts of the body. If you were to have an injury that caused pressure or strain to, say, the sixth and seventh vertebrae in your neck, your wrists and fingers could be affected, as the nerves extending from this area of the spine serve those body parts.

The spinal cord itself ends several inches above the waist. From that point on, individual nerve fibers continue down the spinal canal to their ultimate destinations. Several of the nerves that exit the spinal canal in the sacrum form the *sciatic nerve,* the largest nerve in the body. Irritation of this nerve is responsible for sciatica, as explained on page 6.

## Causes of Back Pain

### *Number-One Cause: Mechanical Disorders*

One autumn morning as Sylvia reached into the trunk of her car to lift a bag of groceries, she felt a sudden excruciating jab of pain in her lower back. Seconds later she was on the ground on her hands and knees, unable to straighten up. She called out for her husband, who picked her up, put her in the backseat of the car, and drove her to the chiropractor.

Sylvia, like so many other backache sufferers, wasn't doing anything unusually strenuous when the pain struck. Her back pain had been waiting for the moment when her weakened muscles would give out.

We've already noted that muscle strain, which is the result of poor posture or incorrect movement and use of the spine, is responsible for about 80 percent of all backaches. If you have poor muscle tone and strength in your extensor and flexor muscles, virtually every move you make has the potential to result in back pain. If you strengthen these muscles, virtually every move you make can keep your back healthy and pain-free. Once you experience back pain, chances are good you will get it again . . . and again . . . and again—unless you make the necessary adjustments in your behavior. Natural therapies and exploration of the mind-body connection can help you on both counts.

What mechanical disorders are responsible for back pain when back and abdominal muscles and ligaments are weak or stressed? Generally they can be classified as strain, sprain, spasm, poor posture, a disk or facet problem, or tension.

### STRAIN

A muscle *strain* occurs when you overstretch or overuse muscles or ligaments. The resulting pain may be confined to a small area of the back or spread out over the spine. Strains can be first-degree (microscopic injury to the muscles), second-degree (macroscopic injury), or third-degree (complete disruption of the muscle), which Sylvia experienced. Regardless of the degree of strain, some individuals can continue to be active for several hours after a strain occurs. After a night's sleep, however, they awaken to moderate to severe pain and stiffness. Every back strain is unique; therefore some movements may not hurt at all, whereas others may be extremely painful.

### SPRAIN

Another common back problem is a *sprain,* which involves partial tearing of ligaments. As you will see in the next chapter, where we discuss diagnosis, back strain and sprain are the most common causes of back pain, yet they are difficult to identify clinically because neither one usually shows on X rays. Whiplash is a specific type of sprain that is mostly confined to the cervical-spine area. People who experience a strain or sprain are at high risk of recurrence of pain and possible chronic pain.

### SPASM

A *spasm* is a sustained involuntary muscular contraction and is actually a good thing. Why? It is like a stop sign: a way the body protects itself from further harm. When muscles are fatigued, weak, or diseased, they may go into spasm and thus prevent any further overstretching or contraction from occurring. The erector spinae muscles are those most commonly affected.

### HERNIATED DISK

Weak muscles can also contribute to a *herniated* or *ruptured disk* (erroneously called a slipped disk since nothing actually slips). If a disk is weakened by age or lack of

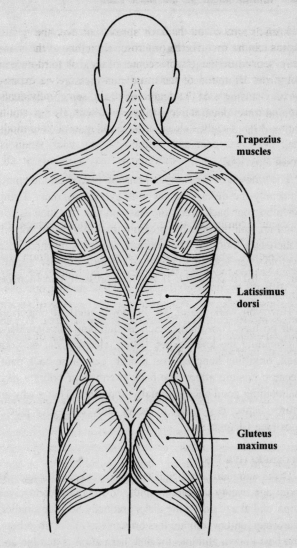

**Trapezius muscles**

**Latissimus dorsi**

**Gluteus maximus**

**I-3 Superficial back muscles**

adequate exercise and the back muscles are not strong, lifting an object incorrectly or lifting something that is too heavy can cause the jellylike center of the disk to rupture or bulge out of the disk wall and put pressure on nearby nerves, causing pain. The pain may be sharp and debilitating and travel down the leg. In some individuals the pain is dull and increases in intensity the more they move around.

## POOR POSTURE

The amount of pressure and tension placed on the spine, especially the disks, changes with every movement. Lying down on your back exerts the least amount. As soon as you stand up, you increase the pressure threefold; when you sit, it increases fourfold. The pressure increases by more than fivefold when you lift an object of medium weight—assuming you lift it correctly. If not, the pressure can increase tenfold.

How you walk, stand, sit, lie down, and lift objects is your posture. Poor habits, such as slumping the shoulders, not bending the knees when lifting, sleeping flat on your back, or sitting hunched over a desk, can cause back pain. Because posture affects the back twenty-four hours a day, maintaining good habits is vitally important. That's why an entire chapter is devoted to better daily back-care guidelines (see Chapter 3).

## DEGENERATIVE DISK

Disks automatically begin to grow weaker with age: At about age twenty the blood supply to the disks themselves stops, and at age thirty, the disks gradually become smaller, lose water, and overall are less effective as shock absorbers. The best known antidote for disk herniation is aerobic and flexibility exercises, which help keep the disks lubricated and promote blood flow around the area.

## MUSCLE TENSION

Back pain associated with stress and tension usually affects the neck, shoulders, and upper back, or the *psoas* muscle, which runs from the front of the lumbar spine and attaches to the thighbone. Emotional and mental stress may also lead to back pain by causing the disks to swell. According to Augustus A. White, M.D., orthopedic surgeon-in-chief at Beth Israel Hospital in Boston, Massachusetts, there is speculation that changes in body chemistry that occur during mental stress may cause the center of the disk, which is largely water, to swell, producing pain.

## FACET SYNDROME

Michael had swung a golf club thousands of times, but one day while practicing for an upcoming tournament the sudden twist sent a jolt of pain through his lower back. He had sprained one of his facet joints, bony structures that line up evenly with those above and below each other and that allow us to bend and twist with minimal friction. The facet joints are held in place by ligaments and are surrounded by synovial tissue, which secretes a lubricating fluid that keeps the joints moving smoothly. When the synovial tissue becomes inflamed, as it does with arthritis or when it is subject to stress, the result is often back pain. In Michael's case the repeated stress of swinging a golf club—as well as his sedentary job during the week—contributed to the sprain. Occasionally the joints may fracture if abnormal tension is placed on them, as when you lift or strain with your back arched.

## *Diseases Associated with Back Pain*

A small percentage of back pain—about 20 percent—is either directly associated with a disease or it can be attributed to a particular physical condition (such as pregnancy), emotional state, or referred pain from a condition elsewhere in the body. Below are the more common diseases associated with back pain.

## OSTEOARTHRITIS

The number-one joint disease is osteoarthritis, a chronic, noninflammatory condition that develops slowly and causes increasing joint pain, stiffness, limited movement, and deformity. Other common names for this disorder are degenerative arthritis and degenerative joint disease. The causes of osteoarthritis are complex, but a brief explanation can help you to understand the reasons behind the back pain that accompanies it.

The cartilage (a stiff body tissue that forms the disks between the vertebrae) undergoes biochemical and metabolic changes as we age, one of which is its tendency to retain excess water. This weakens the structure, or matrix, of the cartilage. The matrix may also be disrupted by tiny fractures that occur over time as the joints are placed under daily stress. These and other factors cause the cartilage to wear away, and place abnormal stress on the surface of joints. This wearing away most often affects the facet joints in the lumbar spine, the most common location of osteoarthritis in the back.

Although some people with osteoarthritis of the facet joints do not have back pain, at least in the early stages, others experience discomfort in the lower back or have pain that travels down one or both legs. Common symptoms include pain over the joints in the lower back, stiffness in the back that lasts about thirty minutes when first getting up in the morning, and limited motion of the spine. As osteoarthritis progresses, symptoms of spinal stenosis become more common: Back pain as well as pain in the buttock, leg, or thigh when standing or walking usually occurs. Many patients have pain in both legs, and some also experience numbness, weakness, and tingling in the legs.

## SPINAL STENOSIS

Larry had been experiencing pain in his right leg and stiffness in his back in the morning for more than a year before numbness in his left leg prompted him to see his doctor. A magnetic resonance imaging (MRI) scan (see Chapter 2, page 35) identified his problem as spinal stenosis, a narrowing of the spinal canal.

Larry also had osteoarthritis, which had caused degeneration of the facet joints and changes in the disks and soft tissue in the affected area. Osteoarthritis is the most common cause of spinal stenosis, but it can also be inherited or caused by an injury or poor posture. The amount of back pain and what other areas of the body are affected depend on which nerves are pressed on in the spinal cord.

## SWAYBACK

The military stance—chest out, shoulders back, stomach tucked in, and buttocks protruding—is believed by many doctors to be a significant factor in back pain. Known as swayback (or lordosis), this posture can aggravate back pain in people with disk disease, osteoarthritis, or other diseases of the facet joints.

## SCOLIOSIS

A healthy, normal spine appears straight when viewed from the front or back; one affected by scoliosis twists to the side (see Figure I-4). This "turn" can develop because of abnormal development of the muscles and bones of the spine ("true" scoliosis) or because of factors not directly associated with the spine ("functional" scoliosis). True scoliosis typically occurs at about age ten, when children begin to undergo a growth spurt. In the area affected by scoliosis, the facet joints are not parallel and the soft tissue shortens. This can cause limited movement in the spine as well as pain in the lower back during certain stretching or bending motions. Most patients, however, are pain-free.

Except for a rare type of inherited infantile scoliosis, the reason for most true scoliosis cases remains a mystery. A popular theory is that some people inherit the tendency for this unbalanced growth, which usually stops once teenagers reach adult height. Most adults with scoliosis have mild

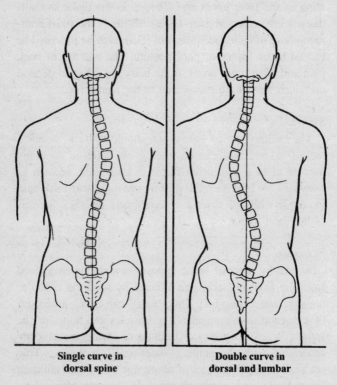

Single curve in
dorsal spine

Double curve in
dorsal and lumbar

I-4   Scoliosis

cases. The experts are divided on the question as to whether adults with scoliosis are more prone to back pain than those without the disorder.

Functional scoliosis can be caused by a difference in leg length or by back spasms. If one leg is shorter than the other, the body compensates by tilting the pelvis to one side and curving the spine to balance the tilt. Even if the legs are of equal length, scoliosis can develop when people consistently favor one side when walking. Back-spasm scoliosis occurs when an injury or disk herniation causes the muscles on one side of the spine to go into spasm.

## KYPHOSIS

An abnormal forward curvature of the spine is called kyphosis, also known as hunchback or roundback. It is less common than scoliosis but can be more severe. Like scoliosis and swayback, it usually develops in childhood and adolescence and is typically an inherited condition or the result of infection or injury. Intermittent back pain is common, although teenagers with mild curvature may not have any pain. Once adolescents stop growing, the pain often ceases, yet stiffness and loss of mobility in the affected area of the spine remain. Kyphosis in adults can be caused by osteoporosis, ankylosing spondylitis, and osteochondrosis of the spine (a degenerative bone condition).

## SPONDYLOLYSIS AND SPONDYLOLISTHESIS

Sometimes a defect in a facet joint causes the vertebra to become loose. The cause may be a birth defect; trauma, such as a fall; a structural weakness in the bone, such as a tumor; or overuse. This condition is called spondylolysis, and mild cases are usually not painful. Over time, stress and strain on the muscles and ligaments that hold the defective vertebral body (composed of a vertebra, its facet joints, and disk) in place may weaken and allow the vertebral body to slide forward and pinch the nerves. This condition is called spondylolisthesis. Back pain associated with either of these conditions occurs in the lower back, back of the thigh, and lower leg and is characteristically an ache, which can be severe, rather than a sharp or shooting pain.

### ARTHRITIC DISORDERS

Diseases that cause inflammation of the joints can affect the spine and result in back pain and limited movement. The most common of these are spondylitis (degenerative arthritis), rheumatoid arthritis, and ankylosing spondylitis. These are considered to be autoimmune diseases, which means the body's immune system attacks its own tissue.

### SPONDYLITIS

This is a fancy name for normal wear and tear in the spine. Although everyone undergoes this process with age, not everyone has pain as a result of it. When people say they know it's going to rain because their back is aching, they likely have spondylitis. Other signs of spondylitis include back pain that is worse after inactivity, pain in the spine after prolonged sitting, and limited ability to turn, twist, or bend the full range of movement of the back.

### ANKYLOSING SPONDYLITIS

*Ankylosing* means "stiffening," so this disease involves both inflammation and stiffening of the spine. Ankylosing spondylitis typically begins when men and women are in their twenties and progresses over years. The pain, inflammation, and stiffness usually start in the lower back and sacroiliac joints, travel up the spine, and destroy the fibro-cartilage in the disks. These areas heal with scar tissue that turns to bone, which causes the vertebrae to fuse together. Some people experience minimal stiffness and pain, while others become permanently bent over and must learn to control constant pain.

## RHEUMATOID ARTHRITIS

This painful inflammatory disease of the joints is one of the few back problems that can be life-threatening. It usually affects the hands, wrists, elbows, feet, hips, and knees, and eventually settles in the spine, where it typically attacks the neck area first. Rheumatoid arthritis causes irreparable damage to the joints and nearby tissues. In severe cases it can destroy the top joint of the spine and cause the vertebrae to slide into the spinal cord and sever it. Approximately 1 to 3 percent of Americans have rheumatoid arthritis. Three times more women than men are affected. Although the cause of rheumatoid arthritis is unknown and there is no cure, the disease and pain can be kept under control.

## TUMORS AND INFECTIONS

Infections that cause back pain are uncommon, yet they are worth mentioning. Sources of infection that can cause back pain include any penetrating wound or open fracture, surgery, a boil that spreads bacteria into the bloodstream, and chronically infected gums and teeth. Infections of the kidneys and bladder can spread to the spine, and people with diabetes are susceptible to all types of infections.

Tumors—new growths of abnormal tissue—are extremely rare causes of back pain, probably less than one in ten thousand. They can affect any part of the spine—ligaments, nerves, muscles, bone, or synovial tissue—and can be either malignant (cancerous) or nonmalignant (noncancerous). Unlike back pain associated with a disk, which is usually relieved by inactivity and rest, the pain caused by tumors is generally continuous and, if the tumor is malignant, gets worse with time. X rays, a CT or MRI scan, or other diagnostic tests are needed to make a positive diagnosis.

## FIBROMYALGIA

People with fibromyalgia experience a general chronic aching pain and tenderness in many areas, including the lumbar spine, inner knee, shoulders, and elbows. This is accompanied by chronic fatigue and muscle soreness. The American Rheumatism Association Committee on Rheumatologic Practice estimates that more than 10 million Americans have this disorder, whereas other authors are more conservative. The chronic pain and fatigue characteristic of this disease typically prevent people from functioning to their potential and contribute to depression. Fortunately this disease responds to a natural healing approach.

## OSTEOPOROSIS AND OSTEOMALACIA

These two bone diseases both involve the loss of bone mass. It is estimated that 29 percent of women and 18 percent of men between the ages of forty-five and seventy-nine have osteoporosis. Osteoporosis usually appears in the axial skeleton, femoral neck, and pelvis. In this disease the bone mineral content and bone matrix remain normal as the bones become porous, similar to Swiss cheese. Loss of bone mass is not painful; however, it leaves the bones in a weakened condition, susceptible to fracture. Many of the fractures may be minute and painless; others may be significant and result in pain and deformity.

In osteomalacia, which is an abnormality of bone mineralization, the bone mineral content and bone matrix decrease. Unlike osteoporosis, people with osteomalacia in the axial spine experience back and bone pain even without having fracture. The pain typically starts in the lower back and then spreads upward.

## FRACTURES

Although the thought of fracturing your back sounds serious, many people are walking around with tiny fractures in their spine and don't even know it. More serious fractures may occur on the vertebral end plates, which usually causes severe pain that gradually decreases over two to three weeks. Once back fractures are healed, most people find they can return to their former level of functioning without pain. Such individuals, however, are especially strong candidates for back-strengthening activities that can avert future back problems.

### *Miscellaneous Factors*

Included in this category are factors and conditions that indirectly cause back pain.

## PREGNANCY

The shift in the center of gravity that occurs in women during pregnancy places a great deal of stress on the lumbar spine. Pregnant women also lose much of their control of the abdominal muscles, placing their back in further distress. Fortunately, except for avoiding medications and back surgery, pregnant women can safely try most other therapeutic approaches to relieve back pain.

## OBESITY

Like pregnancy, obesity shifts the center of gravity forward, placing additional tension and stress on the lower back. Many obese individuals find that once they lose weight, their back problems disappear or decrease significantly.

## OTHER DISEASES AND CONDITIONS

Peter occasionally experiences deep pain in the upper lumbar spine area when his ulcer acts up. Grace always gets lower back pain whenever she is constipated. These and many other diseases and conditions can trigger back pain that is completely independent of any activity or condition that causes true pain in the spine. For example menstruation; inflammation or ulceration of the large intestine; prostate disease; infected fallopian tubes; endometriosis; and cancer of the kidney, bladder, prostate, or rectum are all possible—but remote—causes of back pain. Back pain associated with these diseases tends to be felt deep within the back and to be unaffected by physical activity. Arthritis, infection, or a tumor of the hip can also cause back pain, with accompanying pain in the groin. Individuals with vascular disease, such as atherosclerosis, sometimes experience worsening back pain and deep pain or pins and needles in the legs when they walk.

### PSYCHOLOGICAL

The mind plays a large role in pain and its perception and is discussed in Chapter 4. Here I want briefly to point out two links between mind and back pain. First, backache, like headache or insomnia or getting a cold, is the physical response some people have to emotional stress. For them the back is their Achilles heel—the weak spot in their body that is most affected by tension. Second, while it's true that having back pain can make you feel depressed, it is also true that some severely depressed people have back pain, even though no physical reason can be found. Psychiatric counseling is the best approach for these individuals.

## Healing Back Pain . . . Naturally

There are a multitude of therapies for the many causes of back pain. The natural therapies presented in Part II of this book are listed in alphabetical order; we can also look at them as they are grouped according to similar and shared characteristics. Following are the categories and specific therapies covered:

- **Movement Therapy.** Unlike all the other categories, which have several or more entries, movement therapy is its own group. Muscle strain or functional disorder is the primary reason for backache, and most physicians agree that physical conditioning is of primary importance in any back-care program to help alleviate, prevent, and eliminate the pain. Movement therapy for individuals with back pain is designed to help them to (a) develop or regain sufficient flexibility of the soft tissues, and (b) develop or regain adequate strength of the muscles associated with back function.

- **Relaxation and Stress Reduction Therapies.** These include biofeedback, breathing, hypnosis, massage, meditation, tai chi, visualization, and yoga. The therapies in this category are the ones most intimately associated with the mind-body connection, and they can be very effective as coping and pain-relief techniques for people with chronic back pain.

- **Body-Awareness Therapies.** Postural and realignment therapies, including the Alexander Technique, the Feldenkrais Method, Hellerwork, and Trager therapy, are body reeducation tools you can use to bring your body to a state of balance, better flexibility, and increased muscle tone and strength.

- **Manipulation Therapies.** Manipulation can be of the physical body, as with chiropractic, osteopathic, craniosacral therapy, and Fold and Hold; of the energy surrounding the body, as with therapeutic touch; and of both, as in polarity therapy. All are methods of pain relief. Other therapies that could fall into this category but specifically involve the use of pressure points are given below.

- **Pressure-Point Therapies.** Acupuncture, acupressure, myotherapy, and reflexology are considered pressure-point therapies. Basically you or a practitioner can provide pain relief by using needles, pressure, or massage to release tension and blocked energy in the muscles.
- **Nutritional, Herbal, and Homeopathic Therapies.** These therapies are grouped together because they provide nourishment for the body and spirit. A nutritionally sound diet and weight control have a significant effect on backache, and the benefits of vitamin therapy are a topic for debate. Both homeopathy and herbal medicine can play many roles in the treatment of backache related to muscle strain, including reduction of pain, stress, and muscle tension; removal of toxins from muscles and joints; improvement of blood circulation; and correction of vitamin deficiencies.
- **Physical Therapies.** The use of cryotherapy, thermotherapy, special devices (braces, corsets, cervical collars), traction, and gravity inversion are included in this category of pain-relief methods. These approaches are typically used to relieve pain and increase physical functioning.

# CHAPTER TWO

# Where Do You Turn for Help?

Your back hurts and you feel helpless. Whom should you turn to? Do you need a doctor, or can you handle treatment yourself? What can a doctor do for you that you can't do for yourself? What can natural-medicine practitioners and techniques do for you? How can you prevent the recurrence of back pain?

This chapter answers these questions and gets you on your way to a healthier, pain-free back. The first step is to get a dialogue going with your back and determine whether your pain is an indication of a serious medical problem.

## Do I Need a Doctor?

On Monday morning Karen felt a sharp jab in her lower back when she bent over to pick up her two-year-old son. The pain was annoying, but she managed to play one game of tennis that night. The next morning she woke up with pain and stiffness in the same location. She took ibuprofen, applied light massage, and was mindful of how she lifted and moved for the rest of the day. For the next few days she continued with the same routine—ibuprofen, massage, caution—and by the weekend she stopped the medication.

Ed is a computer programmer who spends at least forty hours a week sitting in front of his computer terminal. Six months ago he began a major project that has kept him not only working longer hours but also under a great deal of stress. The pressure has taken its toll on his back, and for the last four months he has had chronic pain, which he tries to control with medication. Stress reduction techniques, a more "back-friendly" chair, and acupressure would likely provide him with significant relief.

Steven noticed a dull ache in his lumbar spine during one of his daily brisk walks to and from his office. The pain grew progressively worse over a two-week period until one morning he let out a sneeze and suddenly felt a sharp pain shoot down his left leg. Concerned, he contacted his doctor, who performed a thorough examination, magnetic resonance imaging tests, and made a diagnosis of herniated disk.

Most people experience back pain for reasons similar to Karen and Ed's: strain, stress, overuse, and tension. Such backaches usually clear up within a few weeks if common sense is used, and a doctor's visit generally isn't necessary. Some people, however, want the peace of mind of a doctor's opinion, and if you need reassurance, by all means, make an appointment. Fear of the unknown can augment pain as well (see Chapter 4).

Steven, however, displayed one of the signs indicating the need for medical intervention: a sharp, shooting pain in one or both legs (or in one or both arms). Other circumstances that accompany back pain that should prompt you to call your physician include the following:

- Numbness in a leg, foot, arm, or hand.
- Weakness in a leg, foot, arm, or hand.

- Difficulty urinating or defecating, or inability to control these functions.

  Back pain accompanied by any of these conditions could indicate that something—a herniated disk or a tumor, for example—is pressing against the nerves leading to the affected part of the body.

- Dragging a foot when walking. This usually occurs because of a ruptured disk or a compressed nerve that does not allow the leg muscles to raise up the toes.

- Severe back and leg pain accompanied by fever that is not associated with a cold or flu.

- Severe back and/or leg pain that doesn't improve after three to five days' bed rest and two to three weeks of self-care.

- Back pain that wakes you up in the middle of the night.

- Severe back pain that is preceded or accompanied by pain elsewhere in the body or by involuntary weight loss.

- A backache that lasts for more than two weeks. This doesn't always mean there is something seriously wrong; like Ed the computer programmer, failure to practice good back-care techniques can aggravate back pain even though no back disease is at the root of it. A general recommendation for lingering back pain, however, is to have it checked by a physician.

Any of these circumstances could be a signal that there is an infection, fracture, tumor, or other medical problem. Remember, however, that only about 5 to 10 percent of back pain is caused by such medical conditions, and most can be treated successfully using a combination of therapies without surgery.

## The Clinical Examination/Evaluation

The examination referred to in this section is typical of that done by medical doctors, including osteopaths. Specific information about the types of examinations conducted by other health care providers, such as chiropractors and various therapists, are discussed in Part II in the sections that explain their respective therapies.

### *Whom to See*

Many people first contact their family doctor, who most likely fits into one of the following categories:

#### GENERAL PRACTITIONERS

True to their name, these physicians are consulted for general health problems and do not specialize in a particular body system or condition. They will conduct an initial examination, and if they find any indication that further testing is needed, they refer patients to a specialist. General practitioners are gradually being replaced by family physicians. Training for general practitioners includes four years of medical school and a year's internship.

#### FAMILY PHYSICIANS

These individuals are trained to care for all family members, regardless of age. Family physicians receive two additional years of training beyond their internship.

#### INTERNISTS

These physicians specialize in the diagnosis and medical, nonsurgical treatment of the internal organ systems and diseases such as cancer and arthritis in adolescents and adults. Internists study for an additional two years beyond internship.

OSTEOPATHS

Doctors of osteopathy (D.O.s) emphasize the role of the musculoskeletal system—muscles, bones, ligaments, tendons—and the use of spinal manipulation in health and disease. They receive the same amount of training as do medical doctors and spend four years in osteopathic college before their internship or residency.

Some people prefer to choose a medical specialist or may be referred to one by their general or family doctor. *Neurosurgeons* perform surgery involving the brain and the nervous system. For back patients they operate on those with sciatic pain, nerve entrapment, or other nerve problems. *Rheumatologists* are internists who concentrate on treating the many forms of arthritis. *Physiatrists* are physicians who use physical-therapy techniques such as exercise, traction, heat and cold therapy, and TENS to treat and rehabilitate injured and handicapped individuals. *Orthopedists* or *orthopedic surgeons* are specially trained to treat diseases and injuries related to the musculoskeletal system.

## *Tell It Like It Is*

When you visit your doctor, be prepared to help her or him determine the cause of your back pain and the best way to treat it by providing the following information:

- *Characteristics of the pain:* sharp, dull, ache, burning, throbbing, jabbing
- *Pain patterns:* Is the pain constant or does it come and go? If it is transient, what is the pattern? Does it only occur at specific times of the day and/or night? Remember, back pain that wakes you up at night can be a sign of a serious infection or a tumor.
- *Back-pain history:* What previous bouts of back pain have you had, what were they like, and how long did they last?

- *Pain relief:* Does your back pain improve when you exercise? lie down? sit? Which position is most comfortable?
- *Worsening pain:* What causes your back to feel worse? Exercise, coughing, sneezing, sitting, lifting, bending, standing, straining on the toilet, walking?
- *Other symptoms:* Do you have numbness, tingling, weakness, or pain in your legs, feet, arms, or hands? Is your back stiff when you get up in the morning? How long does it last? Have you had any trouble with urination or defecation?

### Diagnosing Your Back Pain

When Naomi visited her family doctor during her first bout of back pain, he asked her to walk up and down the hall, walk on her heels and then on her toes, and to bend and twist her spine in all directions. When she could not walk on her toes, the doctor had a clue that something was pressing on the nerve that ran up the back of her lower leg.

These and other tests physicians do to help them categorize and diagnose back pain are simple, yet they can provide important information. Several techniques are used to determine if something is pressing on a nerve root. For example doctors use a small rubber hammer to test reflexes in the knee and ankle. They also test for numbness by touching various parts on the skin with a pin, cotton swab, or other object while you close your eyes. Where numbness occurs is a clue as to which nerve is being compressed in the spine. Another is the straight-leg-raise test, for sciatica. While you lie on your back, the doctor will slowly raise your legs, one at a time, keeping your knee straight. If you feel pain before the leg reaches a 90-degree angle, it indicates sciatica.

If these or any other test results suggest an abnormality and your back pain falls into the small minority that does not appear to be caused by muscle strain, the doctor usually orders X rays. X rays can reveal problems with bone, such as narrowed disk spaces, bone loss, crushed or misaligned vertebrae, and curvature of the spine. They do not show muscles, tissues, and disks. To see these structures and to test further, the doctor may schedule any of the following tests:

- *Blood work:* to detect infection or disease.
- *Urinalysis:* to rule out a kidney problem. Back pain commonly accompanies kidney infections or kidney stones.
- *CT (computed tomography) scan:* to detect abnormalities in bone, nerves, and soft-tissue structures such as disks. CT emits less radiation than conventional X rays. Some CT scans are done with a relatively harmless injectable dye that allows the structures to be detected better. This dye contains a type of iodine that can cause reactions in people who are allergic to shellfish.

  A CT scan takes approximately thirty to forty-five minutes to complete. You will lie on a table that slides inside a body-scanning unit. A computer-controlled scanner moves above your body and takes many X rays of your back. You will need to lie perfectly still, but there is no discomfort. If you are claustrophobic, ask the doctor or nurse for a mild sedative before the procedure begins.

- *MRI (magnetic resonance imaging) scan:* to detect problems in bone, disks, nerve, and other soft-tissue structures. Unlike CT, which uses radiation to image the body, MRI uses a magnetic force along with a computer. Both CT and MRI can scan the same structures; however, MRI is better able to scan through bone. It cannot be performed on women who have an

IUD or on individuals who have a pacemaker or metal implants such as artificial hips or pinned fractures. Dental implants and fillings are not a problem.

During the procedure, which takes approximately forty-five minutes, you will lie on a table that slides inside the scanning device. The scanner uses magnetic-field and radio energy to produce images of your back. A mild sedative can help if you are claustrophobic.

- *EMG (electromyogram):* to determine if there is muscle or nerve damage. Tiny needles are used to prick the skin along the leg or arm to test if muscle signals and nerve impulses are normal.
- *Bone scan:* to look for "hot spots," areas in the bone where fracture or infection may have occurred. The test itself is painless, although a radioactive dye is injected into the bloodstream. A special instrument detects problem areas in the bone, which show up as black spots on the image.
- *Diskogram:* to show disk damage. A dye is injected into the disk suspected of causing the pain and an X ray is taken. If the disk is normal, the X ray will show that the fluid has not escaped. A herniated disk, however, will allow the fluid to leak out into the surrounding area. This procedure is painful because it reproduces the reason the pain has occurred, yet it is valuable in solving difficult cases.

## After the Examination Is Over

Chances are the diagnosis was strain, sprain, tension, spasm, or perhaps a combination. The doctor most likely gave you the prescription handed out to the majority of people in your situation: Take an anti-inflammatory such as ibuprofen or aspirin, stay off your feet or relax for a few days, and begin strengthening exercises immediately thereafter. This advice is dispensed with the caveat that if the back pain doesn't improve with drugs and rest after a few days, you should return to the doctor.

In any event you can now take matters into your own hands if you so choose. This may mean you decide to forgo the recommended pain medication for an alternative pain-control method, such as hypnosis or visualization. Or you may be thinking, "Okay, along with the medication, I think I'll try _____ ." (This book helps you fill in the blank.) You may even be thinking ahead because you may want to prevent the pain from ever happening again.

The chart that introduces parts II and III can launch you into new realms of therapies. First, however, let's look at the risk factors for back pain and see which ones may have contributed to your pain.

## Risk Factors

The risk factors listed below are those associated with back problems. Several of them you cannot change—heredity, age, and sex—but there is much you can do about the rest.

### Heredity

Several back problems seem to run in families, the most common being intervertebral disk disease and spondylolisthesis (or slipped vertebrae). There is also evidence that herniated-disk problems are hereditary. This may be related to an inherited chemical abnormality in the disks that causes them to fragment or shift position and press against nerves. About a dozen other diseases, all rare, are also associated with back pain. Even if back pain is inherited, movement therapy can be helpful.

## Age and Sex

Back pain is most prevalent among people between the ages of thirty and fifty-five years. Beginning at about age thirty, the disks start to lose fluid and become dry, which makes them more likely to shift and cause pain. Once men reach fifty, they generally have less back pain, whereas women have more, which is associated with the increase in osteoporosis that also occurs in women at this time (see "Osteoporosis," page 24). Women are four times more likely than men to have degenerative spondylolisthesis, a type of arthritis of the lower back. Women also commonly experience back pain during pregnancy, when their center of gravity shifts forward, placing stress on the back.

## Posture

The way you stand, sit, sleep, walk, lift, and carry objects, and otherwise move is your posture. To evaluate whether your posture is causing or contributing to your back pain, try this test. It works best if you wear form-fitting or no clothing. Stand sideways in front of a full-length mirror. Turn your head—but not your body—and look at your image in the mirror. Imagine you have dropped a weighted string down from the center of your head through to your feet. If you have proper posture, the line should pass through the front of your earlobe, the front of your shoulder, the center of your hip, just behind your kneecap, and in front of your ankle bone. When seated, the line should pass through the same spots.

To determine whether you stand and walk with good posture, you can check the soles of your shoes. Look at the bottom of a pair of exercise or walking shoes you have worn for at least several weeks. Excess wear on the outer sides of the heels indicates faulty posture.

How you sleep, lift, and carry objects also have a significant effect on your back. Proper posture is such an important factor in a healthy back that an entire chapter is dedicated to helping you achieve and maintain it (see Chapter 3).

### Previous Back Pain

We mentioned this before, but it's worth repeating: Once you experience one episode of back pain, your chances of having a recurrence are three out of five. Barring repeat pain associated with a structural problem, back pain usually returns because of poor posture and bad habits, which are preventable.

### Overweight

Although not all physicians agree that being overweight is a significant risk factor for back pain, most do concur that extra weight carried in the abdominal region is. If an individual has ten extra pounds of weight in the stomach area, for example, the back muscles must exert fifty pounds of force to counteract the downward pull of that weight. Thus the lower back must contend with an extra fifty pounds of pressure every day, regardless of the activity and in addition to other pressures placed on it. Losing weight may not cure back pain, but it can definitely help.

### Exercise

Both lack of exercise and improper exercise are risk factors for back pain. An explanation of exercises designed to strengthen muscles and prevent backaches, as well as what sports and exercises are not recommended, is detailed in Part II under "Movement Therapy."

### Occupation

Your job may be one of the biggest factors in your back pain. For example, if you spend at least half of your working hours driving a motor vehicle, you are three times more likely to have a herniated disk than the average worker. Active workers also need to beware: Those who must lift, pull, or carry heavy objects as part of their job risk developing lumbar disk disease. Sedentary workers are not spared: It is estimated that spending five years at a sedentary occupation places individuals at risk of herniated-disk disease. Those who do repetitive work, such as assembly-line workers, and stand for hours, are at risk for lower back pain.

Each occupation has its own risks. The best ways to deal with the postures and activities required of you on the job are explored in Chapter 3.

### Stress and Tension

The role of emotional stress in causing or contributing to back pain is uncertain, but many physicians believe there is a definite link. Countless reports now show the correlation between the mind and pain (see Chapter 4). Stress can cause muscular tension, which in turn can result in spasms and pain. If you allow physical or emotional stress, or both, to build up over months and years with little or no reprieve, it may lead to chronic back pain, as well as headache, ulcers, hypertension, colitis, depression, insomnia, and other ailments.

### High-Risk Sports Activities

Certain sports are considered to be high-risk for back pain. Golf, jogging, football, downhill skiing, racquetball, tennis, water skiing, dirt biking, and weight lifting are in this category. If you participate in any of these sports and have a back injury, you can expect to have a recurrence of pain unless you take preventive steps. When you incorporate abdominal- and back-muscle strength-building exercises into your daily routine, you can more confidently pursue your sporting activities.

## Smoking

You may wonder how what you take into your lungs could affect your back, but some experts believe there is a connection. Frequent coughing due to smoking can increase the pressure exerted by the disks in the back and cause back pain. Some also argue that the decreased diffusion of nutrients into the intravertebral disks that is caused by smoking contributes to pain. This is still a controversial area.

## Whom Can You Call?

We assume that you have already seen your physician and have ruled out any disease or other medical condition that requires immediate medical intervention. Now you want to heal and eliminate pain, naturally and safely. There are various types of health care professionals and therapists you can turn to for assistance. Turn to Appendix A for a listing of professional organizations that offer referrals and information; check the listings in the Yellow Pages of your local telephone directory under each individual specialty (biofeedback, chiropractic, and so on); ask your family, friends, and coworkers for referrals; or contact a local pain or back clinic. Ask any professional whose help you are seeking about his or her experience, training, or degrees (if applicable). Your back deserves good care.

Let's look at the variety of alternative healing modalities, as we did in Chapter 1:

- **Movement Therapy.** The number-one person to consult here is your physician. Always check with your doctor before embarking on any kind of exercise or movement-therapy program on your own. After you get a physician's approval and guidelines, it's up to you. Arm yourself with the many excellent books and guidelines on exercise and movement therapy (including this book and the accompanying reference list). You may also want to consult a physical therapist or occupational therapist, both of whom can help you develop a personalized exercise program.

- **Relaxation and Stress Reduction Therapies.** Several avenues are open for you here. You may have access to a pain clinic that has biofeedback and other stress reduction programs as part of its overall services, or you may live in a city that has a center dedicated solely to stress reduction or biofeedback. Healing and wellness centers or clinics are becoming more popular and offer a variety of services from massage to breathing therapy, hypnosis, meditation, tai chi, visualization, and yoga. Or you may contact an independent professional hypnotherapist, massage therapist, or individual who practices and teaches relaxation and stress reduction techniques.

- **Body-Awareness Therapies.** Practitioners of the Alexander Technique, the Feldenkrais Method, Hellerwork, and Trager therapy may be found through their professional organizations. Some physical therapists and occupational therapists are certified to do this type of body therapy; always ask which techniques they have been trained to perform. Individuals who practice these body-awareness techniques are truly teachers, for they instruct people on how to achieve and maintain the kind of postures and body habits that can reduce or eliminate the risk of back pain.

- **Manipulation Therapies.** Practitioners of manipulation therapies include chiropractors, osteopaths, craniosacral practitioners, polarity therapists, and therapeutic-touch therapists. Again, there may be some crossover here: Craniosacral therapists are often osteopaths; polarity therapists may also practice acupressure; and chiropractors may be trained acupuncturists. These multitalented individuals have more knowledge at their disposal to help you heal yourself. I also add here the Fold and Hold method—a form of self-manipulation.

- **Pressure-Point Therapies.** Those who practice acupuncture, acupressure, myotherapy, or reflexology can offer pain relief by releasing tension and blocked energy in the muscles and ligaments. They also teach you pain-relief techniques so that you can practice the therapy on yourself and more easily pursue a muscle-strengthening program.

- **Nutritional, Herbal, and Homeopathic Therapies.** Professionals in this category include nutritionists, naturopaths, herbalists, and homeopaths. Whom you consult here depends on what you are looking for. Naturopaths take a holistic view of back pain and can provide nutritional advice, exercise programs, and herbal remedies, while nutritionists are more likely to concentrate solely on food and nutrition. Both can help with weight-control problems and recommend a vitamin regimen.

Although homeopathy is based more on preventing disease rather than treating ailments once they appear, homeopaths can provide many different remedies for the relief of back pain. A homeopath can help you choose a remedy that fits not only the particular type of back pain you are experiencing but also considers your personality and emotional state. An herbalist can also offer symptomatic relief by using a mixture of herbs that complement one another's healing properties. Herbal medicine is not a licensed profession in the United States, and most herbalists are self-taught or have trained or worked with individuals who have studied the field extensively. It is not unusual to encounter osteopaths and nurses who are knowledgeable about herbal medicine.

CHAPTER THREE

# Guidelines for Daily Back Care

In this chapter you'll learn how to be good to your back as you perform everyday, routine activities and tasks. As you become aware of the effect each of these activities has on your back, you can make the necessary adjustments to reduce or eliminate current or future back pain. We also take a look at what happens to your back during pregnancy and how to reduce discomfort during this time. See Figure I-5 for an overview of the amount of pressure exerted on the back during certain activities.

## Standing

When you are in a relaxed, healthy stance, your back has a normal shallow curve and is neither arched nor flexed. This allows the broad pelvic bones to be aligned under the spine and to best support the spinal column. Even if you have strong back and abdominal muscles, standing can be tiring.

Some people have lifestyles or jobs that require them to be on their feet for many hours, such as nurses, sales and

**Pressure on lower back (pounds)**

I-5 Amount of stress on the back caused by various activities. The least stressful activity is lying down: 66lbs. of pressure. All measurements are based on a 150 lb. adult.

| | Pressure | Activity |
|---|---|---|
| | 66 lbs | Lying down |
| | 154 lbs | Standing |
| | 187 lbs | Walking |
| | 198 lbs | Twisting |
| | 220 lbs | Sitting un—supported |
| | 242 lbs | Coughing |
| | 264 lbs | Laughing |
| | 396 lbs | Bent-knee situp |
| | 468 lbs | Lifting, knees bent |
| | 748 lbs | Lifting, knees straight |

grocery clerks, and factory workers. Standing in one spot for hours increases the curvature of the spine and causes the facet joints to compress. Abdominal muscles become fatigued and relaxed, which causes the pelvis to shift. After just a few minutes the vertebrae begin to sink down, which can make the lower back arch.

To lessen this effect, keep the following hints in mind:

- Distribute your weight evenly on both feet and stand tall. If you must stand in one spot for a long time, place one foot on a low ledge or telephone book and alternate. This decreases the stress on the lower back. About every thirty minutes bend your knees and reach down and touch your toes. This helps lubricate your muscles, ligaments, and joints.
- When standing in front of the bathroom mirror to shave, brush your teeth, or apply makeup, bend forward slightly from the hips and keep your back straight.
- The shoes you wear have an important effect on your back. Avoid raised heels: They make your lower back arch and throw your body out of alignment. For protection against hard pavements, wear sneakers or crepe soles instead of leather soles. Where feasible, bare feet or wearing only socks is preferable to sandals and slingback shoes, which decrease contact with the floor and increase muscle tension in the back.

## Sitting

Believe it or not, sitting is very stressful on your lower back and increases the risk of back strain. When you sit, you place one and one-half times more stress on your back than when you walk or stand. When you are recovering from a back-pain episode, sit less and for shorter periods.

When you sit, choose a chair that offers support, such as a straightback chair. If you have a job that requires you to sit for long periods of time, it's critical that you have the right chair. A good office chair has armrests, seat and back adjustments, and the ability to swivel. Another good chair is a kneeling, or balance, chair, which allows you to put your weight on your knees.

To ease the stress of sitting, get up and walk around and gently stretch at least once an hour. Use a rolled-up towel or small pillow for support behind your lower back if needed. Futons, beanbag chairs, and cushioned sofas, and other soft furniture should be avoided.

Here are some general tips for sitting, wherever you are.

- To sit, use your leg muscles to lower yourself to the edge of the seat. Once on the edge, slide your buttocks to the back of the chair.
- Choose a seat that allows you to rest your feet flat on the floor. If not, your back will tend to arch.
- To stand from a seated position, slide to the edge of the chair and lean forward from your hips. Allow your head to lead you up and out of the chair while you keep your back straight.
- If a chair has armrests, use them. They help reduce the weight exerted on your lower spine, and you can use them to help you get out of the chair.
- Keep your knees slightly higher than your hips. You can use a footstool or even a pile of telephone books under your desk. To reduce stress on the lumbar area, alternate feet every ten to fifteen minutes. In an airplane use a piece of carry-on luggage as a footrest.
- Don't slouch. It might feel good for a while, but it places a lot of stress on your back.
- Sit close to your work. Leaning forward also places additional weight and stress on your back.

- To read while seated, hold the book at chest level.
- If you must drive, support your lower back with a rolled-up towel, pillow, or lumbar roll, and hold your arms slightly bent at the elbows. Adjust the seat so that your leg is extended as little as possible. An extended leg causes you to lose the pelvic tilt and can increase sciatic pain.
- Is it okay to cross your legs? Many doctors say it restricts circulation, places uneven stress on the muscles, and can strain ligaments. Other physicians note that it helps maintain the pelvic tilt.
- If you work at a computer, adjust the monitor so that the top of the screen is at eye level. This keeps you from raising or lowering your head when you look at the keyboard and screen.

## Lying Down Sleeping

The position that provides the least amount of stress on the back is lying down. Not all physicians agree, however, on which variation is the best. Some say it's the one that allows the back to return to its natural curve: on your back with a small pillow or rolled-up towel underneath your knees and another pillow beneath your head and neck. Others advocate lying on your side with a pillow between your bent knees to keep them comfortably apart and a semiform pillow beneath your head and neck. In the first position, the raised knees allow the back muscles to relax. This position places less than one third of the pressure on the disks as does any other lying-down position. The second position places about three quarters of the pressure as when standing.

If you find it impossible to sleep in either of these two positions, you can sleep on your stomach. This position, however, causes the back muscles to shorten and can lead to spasm. To prevent this from happening, place a pillow under your midsection and keep one knee bent up to the pillow to eliminate some of the stress caused by the arching of your back.

What kind of mattress or bed is best? Waterbeds are not for everyone; nor are extra-firm mattresses or sleeping on the floor. Generally any mattress that allows you to sleep comfortably and to wake up feeling rested is good for you. If your mattress sags in the middle, it's time to get a new one. Consider your mattress an investment.

Once you are in bed, you can get up and out with minimal pain by using the logrolling method. This approach allows you to reduce any twisting of your body and to use your arms instead of your painful back and abdominal muscles to get out of bed:

1. While lying on your back, roll over on your side toward the edge of the bed. Move your shoulders and hips at the same time—don't twist.
2. Once you are on your side, slowly raise your knees until your feet are dangling over the edge of the bed.
3. Then use your hands and elbow and push against the bed as you bring your legs to the floor. From that position, stand up.

## Bending

When you do tasks that require you to bend and lean, such as filling and emptying the dishwasher, tying your shoes, and vacuuming, let your legs do the work. Here are some tips for some routine activities that require bending:

- To help you reach your feet when putting on socks or tying your shoes, raise one foot onto a stool, chair, or bed. Bend your other knee, lean forward from your hips, and keep your neck and back aligned. Return the foot to the floor and repeat with the other foot. Another approach is to sit down and bend forward from the hips.

- To vacuum, rake leaves, or do other tasks that require you to bend and lean, use your feet as your foundation. Stand with your feet shoulder-width apart and with one foot in front of the other. As you reach forward and vacuum, for example, shift your weight back and forth between your two feet. Remember to bend from the hips to align your torso.
- To reach something low to the ground, such as helping a small child get dressed, squat down, and rest one knee on the floor for support if needed.

## Lifting/Carrying

Whenever you lift a box or an object of medium weight (a weight you can handle normally without straining), the pressure on your disks increases more than five times what it is when you are lying down—and that's if you lift properly! If you lift incorrectly—bending at the waist instead of bending the knees—the pressure increases ten times.

A good general rule to follow is: If you are recovering from a back-pain incident, don't lift anything. Lifting requires the cooperation of back, abdominal, leg, shoulder, arm, and neck muscles. You can strengthen all of these muscles without lifting—see Part II, "Movement Therapy."

The following tips on how to lift objects safely and correctly are for once you are past the acute-injury stage and are healing, and for prevention of future back problems:

- When you lift objects again after a back-pain episode, start with objects that weigh less than you know you can lift. If you begin to feel strained or tired, stop lifting. Sometimes pain doesn't recur until several hours after the lifting is over.

- Leaning over and lifting an object, as when you lift groceries out of a shopping cart or a baby out of a crib, requires careful attention, especially if your back is hurting now. Both shopping carts and cribs encourage people to lift in a potentially harmful way: bent with their knees straight, reaching forward to lift, and then lifting away from rather than close to the body. To lift groceries or a baby safely, position one foot several inches behind the other. Lunge forward as you bend from the hips, lift the object, bring it close to you, and then straighten up. An alternative way is to tighten your abdominal muscles, place one foot up on a footstool or a few telephone books, and lean your forearms on the edge of the cart or crib. As you lift up, bring the package or infant close to your body.

- To lift an object from the floor, stand close to the object and spread your feet wide to give yourself a foundation of support. Bend your knees, keep your back straight, and grasp the object. Hold the object close to your body as you straighten your legs and stand tall.

- When you need to lift and twist, as when retrieving something from the bottom shelf of the refrigerator, squat and pull the object toward you. While in the squat position, twist and then straighten up.

- Avoid lifting an object above your waist. If you need to put something on a high shelf, place one foot on a stool before you reach up. This will help keep your back from arching.

Pocketbooks, briefcases, and luggage are items people carry most often. The secret here is to share or balance the weight.

- A briefcase or pocketbook with a shoulder strap is best because the strap helps distribute the weight to the upper torso. Switch sides frequently to balance the stress placed on the body.
- A pocketbook can also be carried with the strap across the chest. Keep one hand underneath the pocketbook for extra support.
- For optimal balance of weight, two small suitcases are better than one large one. If you must carry one large one, keep your shoulders level and switch sides frequently. You might also consider getting luggage with wheels or using a luggage cart.
- When carrying small items such as books, hold them in front of you close to your body. Backpacks, packed lightly, allow you to distribute the burden evenly. If carrying an infant, use a front-pack carrier, which distributes the baby's weight evenly in front of you.

## Sex

People with back pain often fear that sexual activity will cause damage or more pain. Although it's usually best to avoid sex if you have acute back pain and muscle spasm, in many cases sex is actually helpful, as long as you choose your positions carefully.

During sexual relations both women and men use pelvic motions, which occur through the lower back and the hip joints. Any position that allows you to control these motions, and thus not feel vulnerable, is suggested. Forward motion of the pelvis can ease pain and stress in the lumbar area. A good position recommended by many back specialists is to lie on your side, either facing your partner or lying back to front. An alternative is to be on top during sex. Your partner should be propped up with pillows to allow you to keep a bent-knee position. This tilts the pelvis forward and minimizes stress on the lower back. If the pelvis is "rocked" through its normal range of motion and there is moderate back arching, these motions can actually help to prevent back problems.

Trust and communication between partners are important when dealing with back pain and sex. Having sex during the healing process can certainly be as fulfilling as it is during other times, perhaps even more so because it gives people a reason to take a look at their relationship and each other's feelings.

## Pregnancy

The guidelines discussed in this chapter regarding sitting, standing, bending, lying down, and carrying also apply during pregnancy, but even more so. (See Part II, "Movement Therapy" for exercise tips during pregnancy.) Pregnant women with back problems usually had a somewhat weakened back before they became pregnant; their new temporary condition merely sets off the pain. As the abdomen grows larger, women lean backward and produce greater stress on the lower back. Near the end of the pregnancy the ligaments of the spine are softened by the same hormones that are secreted to prepare the birth canal. The already strained lower back is stressed further and becomes painful.

To prevent or reduce back pain during pregnancy, a daily movement program should be followed. Prenatal exercise classes are also recommended. Consult your physician before starting any type of physical activities while pregnant.

Here are a few general hints to consider during pregnancy:

• Change positions often; prolonged standing or sitting are especially stressful on the back.

- While sitting, do ankle circles to help circulation and shoulder circles to reduce upper back strain.
- While standing, tilt your pelvis by frequently shifting back and forth from one straightened leg to the other.
- As you walk, be conscious of your posture: tilt your pelvis forward, raise your rib cage, stretch the back of your neck, and keep your chin level.

Now that we have explored the physical aspects of back pain, we turn to the mind-body connection.

# CHAPTER FOUR

# The Mind-Body Connection

In recent years *mind-body connection* has become a household phrase. The intimate relationship between emotions and physical reactions and the role that special connection plays in our health and well-being is not new; it is at least as old as humankind itself. Hippocrates, who believed health is a harmonious state that exists among the mind, body, spirit, and the external environment, was certainly aware of it. He knew that "The natural healing force within each one of us is the greatest force in getting well." Natural therapies support this concept because they are based on and work with the mind-body connection. Until recently the wisdom of this Father of Medicine was largely absent from the world of Western medicine; now such notable thinkers and physicians as Deepak Chopra, Norman Cousins, Andrew Weil, Bernie Siegel, Joan Borysenko, among others, are sharing information about mind-body medicine with the general public.

## Understanding the Mind-Body Connection

"Mind and body are inextricably linked, and their second-by-second interaction exerts a profound influence upon health and illness," says Kenneth R. Pelletier, Ph.D., M.D. (hon.), of Stanford University School of Medicine. Deepak Chopra explains the link in more detail: "Mind and body are inseparably one. . . . A basic emotion such as fear can be described as an abstract feeling or as a tangible molecule of the hormone adrenaline. Without the feeling there is no hormone; without the hormone there is no feeling." And Pelletier says that "fear and anger can trigger chain reactions that affect blood chemistry, heart rate, and the activity of every cell and organ system in the body. . . . All of that is now indisputable fact."

Indisputable for some, but not for everyone. Conventional medicine and medical education do not tend to teach students and physicians methods of decreasing or eliminating pain. Instead they focus on diagnosis, surgery, and pharmacology. Much of the research monies, which come mostly from pharmaceutical companies, are spent to develop new drugs or test existing ones.

Conventional medicine definitely plays a critical role in our health care system. Infections, broken bones, tumors, and medical emergencies are usually best handled, at least initially, by conventional approaches. Even in such situations, however, holistic medicine can play a complementary role. When less serious conditions are presented, such as backache, natural therapies can often be the primary or only approach necessary to provide relief.

### The Mind-Body Dialogue

Earlier we mentioned that the mind-body connection allows you to communicate with your body and your pain. This can happen because natural medicine involves an awareness of pain and dis-ease as a part of the self, acceptance of the illness and its symptoms, and then the willingness to accept that there are other influences on the pain, such as emotional and attitudinal changes, behavior modifications, and stress and relaxation.

"When I stopped fighting my back pain and accepted it as a part of me, it was as if I had found a new friend—me!" said Darlene. "Fighting myself was tiring; when I started a dialogue with my pain and turned to natural therapies such as meditation and biofeedback, I immediately felt more confident, more in control of my life and my pain."

People who make lifestyle modifications and adopt holistic therapies into their lives, such as stress reduction and attention to nutrition and exercise, make new discoveries about themselves, their world, and their role in it. Like Darlene, they connect with parts of themselves they had ignored, denied, or taken for granted in the past. Incorporation of natural, holistic behaviors into your lifestyle not only helps heal those areas that may be in dis-ease; it also creates and maintains a state of healthy harmony in your body, mind, and spirit.

## Pain and Emotions: Fear, Anger, Hopelessness

Pain is a wakeup call that something is out of balance or in dis-ease in your body. The pure pain can then be affected, becoming either worse or better, once emotions and judgment come into play. For example, if you tell a four-year-old child that he will get a shot at the doctor's office, he may cry and scream in anticipation of the pain before you even get into the waiting room. But if you calmly explain to him that a gentle, caring person is going to give him some healing medicine through his skin, he will probably only whimper or cry when the needle actually pokes him.

Emotions—we all have a wealth of them, and they guide us in all our tasks and decisions. Each expression of joy or fear, love or anger, is a manifestation of who we are at that particular moment. Emotions such as joy and love, for example, can make people feel invincible; sorrow, fear, and anger, however, can create internal stress, muscle tension, and chemical changes that can cause or worsen back pain. When you "talk" to your body and your pain through the avenue of natural therapies, you gain a different perspective on those feelings. Rather than hold on to the belief that the sadness, anger, or fear you feel is negative or wrong, you can view the feeling as a part of the healing process and in a positive light.

If you feel out of control and hopeless about your back pain, fear is not far behind. Fear is the result of hopelessness. You can get relief for your back pain, but your first step must be to act on the belief that you can do something to improve your situation. It took Henry a while to learn this. Every time Henry's back "went out," he knew he would miss several days of work and quality time with his two young sons, who, like Henry, were avid hikers and rafters. Along with Henry's fear was anger and a sense of helplessness that these back-pain attacks would continue intermittently for the rest of his life.

Henry is like millions of people whose emotions lead them to experience physical symptoms such as increased muscle tension, headache, stomach distress, and other results of stress, which not only augment back pain but also cause people to resort to harmful behaviors. Henry, for example, took large doses of painkillers when a back-pain incident occurred a day before a planned rafting trip. The first day of the trip he became nauseous and faint and had to be brought back home. In his case these symptoms were good: If he had continued in his "painless" (drugged) state, he probably would have harmed himself. Unlike conventional drug treatments for pain, natural treatments are safe and largely without adverse effects. This makes natural therapies firm foundations on which to take the first step toward pain relief.

Although emotions can make pain worse, positive attitudes and emotions can relieve pain. To that end try the following experiment:

1. Rate your back pain from 1 to 10.
2. In your mind's eye, picture a thermometer in front of you, with 0 on the bottom and 100 at the top. How does your pain rate right now—30, 40, 50, or higher? Picture the liquid at the number that corresponds to your pain level.
3. Now imagine you have just had a very frustrating day at work or school; maybe you had an argument with your best friend or spouse or you have overdrawn your bank account. What happens to the liquid in the gauge? It moves up, indicating an increase in pain. Now that you see that stress can increase pain, you can also make it decrease.
4. Push the thoughts about your troubles aside for a moment and picture yourself in a peaceful setting—a deserted beach, a meadow full of flowers, a church. Everything is perfect: the air is clean, the temperature is warm, and no one else is around. What happens to the liquid in the gauge? For many people it goes down. If it stays the same or goes up, something else is probably causing stress in your life. If you can identify the stressor and discuss it, chances are the liquid will go down.

## Dealing with Chronic Back Pain

The definition of *chronic pain* varies, depending on which medical text or physician you talk to. When dealing with backache, it generally means any pain that lingers longer than two months. A significant factor in chronic pain is the part that thoughts, emotions, and other people's responses to you play. According to Dennis C. Turk, Ph.D., director of the Pain Evaluation and Treatment Institute of the University of Pittsburgh School of Medicine, and Justine M. Nash, Ph.D., a psychologist at Miriam Hospital in Providence, Rhode Island, "Perhaps the most vital message . . . is that psychological problems rarely cause pain; but the longer chronic pain exists, the more likely it is that emotional factors are prolonging it." Thus it follows that therapies that focus on resolving these emotional situations can be effective against chronic pain. Some of the most effective natural therapies for chronic back pain are self-treatment strategies such as breathing therapy, self-hypnosis, biofeedback, visualization, and meditation, all of which allow people to have some control over their pain.

Perhaps you have tried one or more of these therapies and had mixed results. Usually the success of these approaches depends on your attitude or on outside circumstances such as lack of support from your family or friends. Often what people lack is patience: Stress reduction techniques do not provide the near-instant relief that drugs can give, but their effects are safe and often long-lasting.

## Ready, Set . . .

What if you want to try more than one holistic therapy at the same time? By all means, do! The majority of natural therapies are not mutually exclusive. In fact it is recommended that you try several at the same time, which will help you experience even more clearly the mind-body relationship.

For example relaxation therapies such as breathing and meditation quiet both the mind and the body and thus are excellent preludes to massage, acupressure, and other physical therapies. Michael discovered this connection when he began meditating every day. "The mental relief I got was great, but what I was really after was relief from the back pain and spasms—and I got it! I didn't believe the mind-body connection would be so strong, but I was wrong." Michael meditates before his acupressure sessions and his daily movement routines because, he says, "it relaxes me and prepares my body for healing."

What's the first thing people do before they start a new project or adventure? They take a deep breath! Breath is the beginning and the foundation of life; it connects the conscious and unconscious. Breathing therapy is explained in detail later in this book, but before you take the plunge into Part II, we want to introduce a simple, basic breathing exercise that, with practice, can quickly put you into a state of deep relaxation.

According to Andrew Weil, M.D., a leading expert on natural and conventional medicine, "The single most effective relaxation technique I know is conscious regulation of breath." The following breathing exercise is one he recommends for everyone. It is the perfect prelude to the rest of this book . . . and the rest of your life.

BREATHING EXERCISE

1. Place the tip of your tongue against the ridge behind and above your front teeth. Keep it there throughout the entire exercise.
2. Exhale completely through your mouth, making a "whoosh" sound.

3. Close your mouth. Inhale deeply and quietly through your nose to the count of 4.
4. Hold your breath for a count of 7.
5. Exhale through your mouth to a count of 8, making a sound.
6. Repeat steps 3, 4, and 5 for a total of four breaths.

Do this breathing exercise in any position that is comfortable for you and maintain good posture: straight back, relaxed neck and shoulders. Practice this routine at least twice a day and whenever you feel stressed or fatigued. During your first month of practice only do up to four breaths at a time, but you can practice as often as you wish. After a month increase to eight breaths each time if you are comfortable with it.

There are many ways to make the connection between mind and body easier to experience and understand. Some of the most effective and common ways are explained in Part II. There are others, and we hope you will feel free to explore beyond the pages of this book.

PART II

# WHICH NATURAL THERAPY SHOULD YOU CHOOSE?

Okay, you're intrigued, or at least curious, about natural therapies. How do you know which therapy to choose? Bernie Siegel, M.D., believes that the most important factor in choosing a treatment strategy is that you have a positive attitude about it and that you believe in it. "Treatment chosen out of fear is unlikely to be helpful," says Dr. Siegel, just as is therapy that is picked because your mother, spouse, or best friend wants you to try it. "The body heals, not the therapy," Siegel explains.

This part of the book gives you an opportunity to learn about some of the many natural ways you can manage back pain. No one treatment can do it all. The recommended strategy for back pain, as with most physical conditions, is a holistic approach that incorporates several methods. As you explore the therapies in this part of the book, keep an open mind. You can always stop doing something that does not appeal to you or help you.

We urge you to explore the therapies in this book. To help you decide which ones are right for you, here are some suggestions:

- Allow your curiosity to lead you to new possibilities. Nearly everyone has an adventuresome part of himself or herself that wants to take a chance and try something new.
- Talk to family, friends, coworkers, and others who have used the therapies you are considering. Ask lots of questions: How did it work? How long until they got relief? How much did it cost? Would they do it again? How did they learn it? Whom did they go to? and so on. Remember that people respond differently to different therapies. What you need is general information to help you make a decision.
- A little apprehension about new things is normal. To help you get beyond it, try guided meditation or visualization. Meditation and visualization tapes are available (see Appendix B) that you can use in the privacy of your own home. If you try these approaches, you will likely find that as your apprehension fades, so will your pain.
- Contact appropriate associations and ask for references and names of local practitioners. See Appendix A for a list of associations and institutions.
- Attend lectures, seminars, and demonstrations. Practitioners and therapists often host free or inexpensive no-obligation events to explain their techniques. These provide excellent opportunities to ask questions and meet other people who may have experienced the therapy.
- Read up! We hope we have piqued your curiosity and empowered you to look farther. "Suggestions for Further Reading," in the back of this book, is a good place to start.

As a visual aid we have prepared the following chart, "Review of Natural and Medical Therapies." To use this chart, go to the far left-hand columns and choose what you want to achieve; then look across the row next to your choice and match up the therapies. For example, if you want to prevent acute back pain, choose "Prevention and Maintenance" under "Acute Pain." On the corresponding row you are referred to Alexander Technique, Diet/Nutrition, Feldenkrais Method, Hellerwork, Movement Therapy, Physical Devices, Polarity Therapy, Tai Chi, Trager Therapy, Yoga, and TENS. Turn to the description of any or all of these therapies: Part II for natural therapies and Part III for medical therapies.

Keep the following definitions in mind when you use the chart. "Treatment" refers to therapy options that are effective in acute or chronic back pain. Some of these therapies can also be used as part of a prevention and maintenance program. Try those that you find appropriate for your situation. "Prevention and Maintenance" includes therapies to help prevent back pain and/or maintain a minimal or pain-free state. These are typically initiated after the first acute pain attack is under some control. "Pain Control" is a nonpharmaceutical approach and includes the therapies mentioned in Chapter 4, "The Mind-Body Connection."

One last suggestion: Go back to the end of Chapter 4 and do the breathing exercise. That should calm any hesitation jitters or apprehensions you have. And then read on!

## ACUPRESSURE

Acupressure is an ancient technique in which pressure is applied, usually with the fingers or hands, to certain points on the body in order to restore the flow of energy, or "vital force," that moves throughout the body. Energy gets blocked at sites of injury or tension. When the energy is freed up, the benefits can include relief from pain, muscle

# REVIEW OF NATURAL AND MEDICAL THERAPIES

| PAIN CONTROL | CHRONIC PAIN | | ACUTE PAIN | | |
|:---:|:---:|:---:|:---:|:---:|:---|
| | Prevention and Maintenance | Treatment | Prevention and Maintenance | Treatment | |
| | | | | | **NATURAL THERAPIES:** |
| • | | | | • | Acupressure |
| • | | • | | • | Acupuncture |
| | • | | • | | Alexander Technique |
| • | | • | | | Biofeedback |
| • | | • | | • | Breathing |
| | | • | | • | Chiropractic |
| | | • | | • | Craniosacral Therapy |
| | | • | | • | Cryotherapy |
| | • | | • | | Diet/Nutrition |
| | • | | • | | Feldenkrais Method |
| | | • | | • | Fold and Hold |
| | | • | | • | Gravity Inversion |
| | • | | • | | Hellerwork |
| | | • | | • | Herbal Medicine |
| | | • | | • | Homeopathic |
| • | | • | | • | Hypnosis |
| | | • | | • | Massage |
| • | | • | | • | Meditation |
| | • | | • | | Movement Therapy (Exercise) |
| | | • | | • | Myotherapy |
| | | • | | • | Osteopathic |
| | • | | • | | Physical Devices |
| | • | | • | | Polarity Therapy |
| | | • | | • | Reflexology |
| | • | | • | | Tai Chi |
| | | • | | • | Therapeutic Touch |
| | | • | | • | Thermotherapy |
| | | | | | Traction |
| | • | | • | | Trager Therapy |
| • | | | | | Visualization |
| | • | | • | | Yoga |
| | | | | | |
| | | | | | **MEDICAL THERAPIES:** |
| | | | | | **DRUGS:** |
| | | • | | • | Analgesics |
| | | • | | | Antidepressants |
| | | • | | • | Muscle Relaxants |
| | | | | | Nonsteroidal anti-inflammatory drugs (NSAIDs) |
| | | | | | **INJECTION THERAPY:** |
| | | • | | • | Analgesic |
| | | • | | | Chymopapain |
| | | • | | • | DMSO |
| | | • | | | Epidural Cortisone |
| | | • | | | Facet Joint |
| | | • | | | Peripheral Nerve Block |
| | | • | | | Sclerosant |
| • | • | | | | SURGERY |
| • | • | • | • | • | TENS |

tension, and stress. This invisible force is called *prana* in Ayurvedic medicine; *kundalini* in yogic philosophy; *ki* in Japanese medicine and martial arts; and *chi* (pronounced "chee" or "key") in Taoist philosophy. All of these terms can be used interchangeably to refer to the vital force.

According to Eastern teachings, the vital force moves throughout the body along twelve channels called *meridians*. Each meridian is associated with a different body system, yet they are all interconnected. Along the meridians are acupressure (or "trigger") points where the meridians reach the skin surface. When pressure is applied to these points, the vital force can be manipulated and balanced, thus relieving tension and muscle strain. Both acupressure and acupuncture (page 80) are based on the same principle of working these points to regain optimum energy flow and balance in the body.

Several other therapies, including shiatsu, Dō-In, and G-Jo, are similar to acupressure in their approach and in the points used for treatment, yet there are some differences. Acupressurists and shiatsu practitioners, for example, vary in how hard and how long they press the points and whether they use one hand or two. Some acupressurists work on the points using their palms, feet, elbows, and even their knees. Generally, however, the procedures among these similar therapies are the same. ("Suggestions for Further Reading" offers several books that describe these and other acupressure techniques in detail.)

## Treating Yourself with Acupressure

You can treat yourself with acupressure once you become familiar with your energy points. We suggest, however, that you first visit a trained, licensed professional so that you can learn firsthand where the points are and how a treatment feels. You might also consider taking an introductory course in acupressure and learn how to treat yourself and perhaps share the healing experience with others.

To find an acupressure point (use Figure II-1 to help you), use one or two fingers and press around the area that feels tense. These points are usually found in muscular areas—and the back has an abundance of muscles. Other acupressure points can be found in joints and areas of bone depressions.

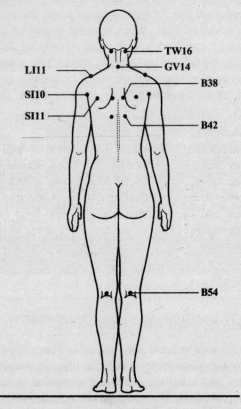

**II-1 Acupressure points for upper back pain**

Once you locate a tight area, you may feel a knot or a tight muscle and also some soreness in the center of it. Soreness is an indication that energy is blocked. From one to several minutes of firm pressure on the painful spot will help release the blocked energy. As you press, the feeling should be somewhere between pleasure and pain. When a blockage is finally released, you will feel a slight pulsing coming from the point. Don't be discouraged if you don't feel the pulse the first few times you do acupressure; it takes practice to become sensitive to all your body has to say. Also, pain relief may not occur instantly. When you press on acupressure points, you stimulate the body's natural tendency to heal. This process takes time, sometimes up to thirty minutes. When applying acupressure to a point that has a mirror opposite—B42, for example, is located on both sides of the spine (see Figure II-1)—you can press on both points simultaneously or one at a time.

For maximum effectiveness acupressure, as well as all the other therapies discussed in this book, should be approached holistically. That is, complement it with one or more other therapies, including movement therapy, herbal remedies, and lifestyle modifications. Also keep in mind that acupressure is not recommended for severe or chronic back problems, such as degenerative disease or a ruptured disk, nor is it meant to replace conventional treatment when it is needed.

## THE MERIDIANS AND CORRESPONDING ORGANS

The abbreviations CV, GV, and so on in the accompanying figures refer to the meridians through which the vital energy flows and connects the acupressure/acupuncture points and the corresponding organs. Acupressurists and acupuncturists use these abbreviations when referring to the pressure points.

| | | | |
|------|--------------------|------|------------------|
| Lu | Lung | LI | Large Intestine |
| Sp | Spleen | St | Stomach |
| H | Heart | SI | Small Intestine |
| K | Kidney | B | Bladder |
| TW | Triple Warmer | P | Pericardium |
| Lv | Liver | GB | Gallbladder |
| CV | Conception Vessel | GV | Governing Vessel |

The Conception and Governing vessels, which run alongside the spinal cord, store energy and are especially important in back pain. Points along these meridians are pressed to strengthen and calm and to increase the results obtained from stimulation of other points along other meridians.

## For Upper Back Pain

Treating your own upper back can be a bit difficult. Here is an opportunity to recycle your old tennis balls. Lie on your back on a mat or on the floor and place a tennis ball or racquetball under the acupressure points. If the balls are too hard, use a soft rubber ball of the same size. Some of the spots you want to reach are TW16, GV14, LI11, SI11, B38, and B42 (Figure II-1). Breathe deeply as you maintain firm but gentle pressure on each point for one to five minutes or until the pain is reduced. While you are pressing on these points, there are others located on the arms that, when held along with those on the upper back, can help unblock the energy: SI10, LI11, and LI10 (see figures II-1 and 2).

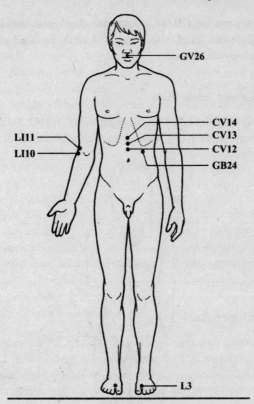

**II-2   Acupressure points for middle back pain**

## For Middle Back Pain

One of the acupressure points that relieves middle back pain is in your foot. Applying pressure to this spot, located in the webbing between your big toe and the adjacent toe (see L3 in Figure II-2), is effective for muscle spasms as well as headache, insomnia, and cramps. Several other acupressure points beneficial for the middle back—GV26, CV14, CV13, CV12, and GB24—are shown in Figure II-2.

Do not press on CV 12, 13, or 14 when your stomach is full. For extra relief, also press B54 while pressing any of the above-named points.

## For Lower Back Pain

Press on points B23 (to the right of B47), B47, B48, and B54 (see Figure II-3). Another special point for lower back

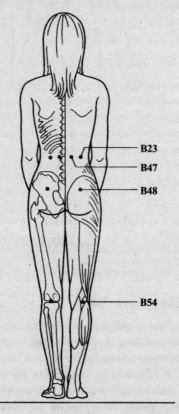

**II-3  Acupressure points for lower back pain**

pain is located four finger widths below the elbow crease of the forearm. To locate it, place all four fingers of one hand together and place them against the elbow crease. The point you want to press is located on the middle of your forearm. When you touch this area, feel for a muscular band and wiggle the middle finger of the arm on which you are looking for the point. If you feel the muscle move, you have found the spot. The point is directly under this muscle, so press directly on it. Hold it firmly for five seconds, then release. Do the same on the other arm.

## Special Points for Back-Pain Relief

Pressing certain points along the Bladder meridian, which governs the back muscles, can bring relief. The points especially helpful in relieving tension and pain in the back are located behind the thighs, the backs of the knees, and in the center of the calves (Figure II-4). You can also press these points while holding other points discussed in the paragraphs above.

## What to Expect from an Acupressure Therapist

If you need help in finding an acupressure therapist or a shiatsu practitioner, consult Appendix A. Prepare for your first visit by wearing comfortable, loose-fitting clothing. You'll be asked about your personal and medical history, and your pulse will be checked. Then it's time for your treatment, which will probably take place on a padded massage or treatment table or on a futon. During a typical one-hour session you may be asked to shift position several times, but it will always be with your comfort in mind. The therapist will "feel" for spots where your life energy is blocked and then press to release the tension. What occurs at that point is what many patients call a good hurt. One or

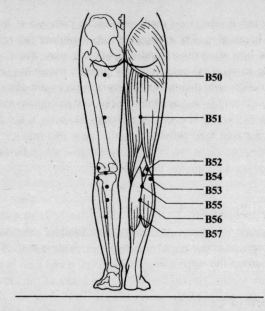

B50
B51
B52
B54
B53
B55
B56
B57

**II-4   Special acupressure points along the Bladder meridian**

more applications of pressure usually release the hurt and allow your energy to flow freely.

Acupressure therapists, like practitioners of other natural disciplines, often recommend dietary changes as part of a self-help program. An eating plan that is free of most or all animal products or a macrobiotic diet are the most popular (see "Diet/Nutrition").

## How Does Acupressure Work?

Western medicine offers several possible explanations. One is the gate-control theory. This theory states that messages from sensory nerves travel faster than pain messages. Thus the sensory impulses reach the brain first and "shut the gate." If you hit your finger with a hammer and immediately rub it, you don't really reduce the pain, yet it feels better because merely rubbing the skin inhibits the pain. This is how acupressure and acupuncture may work, according to some researchers: They provide maximum sensory nerve stimulation to minimize pain stimulation. Another theory is that acupressure (as well as acupuncture) stimulates the release of endorphins, the body's natural neurochemical that inhibits pain.

Or it may well be that the explanation offered by Eastern practitioners is the correct one, that as the life force moves along the meridians, it can become blocked, often because of muscle tension or stress. Acupressure and acupuncture release these barriers and help return your body to a balanced state. (Also see another type of therapy associated with pressure points—"Myotherapy"—which is discussed elsewhere in this section.)

## A Word of Caution

Because acupressure involves the use of pressure and increases blood flow, it should be avoided if you have any of the following medical conditions. Inform your practitioner of all medical situations during your first visit. Properly trained acupressure therapists understand under which circumstances acupressure should not be performed.

- Risk of bleeding or a blood clot.
- Osteoporosis.
- Recent tissue damage, bone fractures, or inflammation. Avoid acupressure in the affected areas.
- Pregnancy. There are some pressure points on the leg that acupressure practitioners say can increase the chance of miscarriage. Of those mentioned above, do not press on LI10 and SI10 when pregnant.
- Epilepsy or high blood pressure.

# ACUPUNCTURE

For more than five thousand years the Chinese have used this medical technique which, like acupressure, is based on the idea of keeping the vital energy in balance. Instead of pressure, however, acupuncture (from the Latin *acus,* "needle" and *punctura,* "to prick") utilizes sharp, thin needles that are inserted into the skin at acupuncture points along the meridians (see "Acupressure," page 69) in order to unblock obstructed energy.

## Acupuncture for Back Pain

Acupuncture is not a do-it-yourself treatment. See Appendix A for information on how to locate an acupuncturist in your area.

There are two main approaches to acupuncture in America. Western practitioners typically ask about symptoms and medical history and then begin treatment. If you go to a medical acupuncturist (an M.D. trained in acupuncture), a physical examination will be conducted as well. There are only about three thousand such professionals in the United States. Contact the American Academy of Medical Acupuncturists (see Appendix A).

Acupuncturists trained in the traditional Chinese practice, however, gather much more information. They observe a person's eyes, skin, face, tongue, and overall appearance. The Chinese believe the texture, color, and shape of the tongue, for example, can reveal where problems may be lurking in the body. They ask about eating habits and elimination problems, and they listen to the voice, breathing, and coughing and note any mouth odor.

Some traditional acupuncturists use *pulse diagnosis,* in which they feel the radial artery pulse in the wrist and, from that, check nine different pulses and identify which areas of the body have a blockage or disturbance. For those not trained in this method, an instrument called a *ryodoraku* can provide similar information. To use this painless method, you simply hold a metal cylinder in the palm of your hand. The acupuncturist uses a pencillike tool attached to a monitoring device to measure the resistance of specific points along the meridians by touching the ryodoraku point to the skin and checking the monitor reading.

The needles, a mere 2¼ to 3½ inches long, are typically made of stainless steel or silver alloy. After the practitioner inserts the needles into the skin—just a few millimeters—they remain there for about twenty minutes. The answer to the inevitable question Does it hurt? is "yes and no." Some people feel little or no pain when the needles are inserted; others say it is a "good hurt," like releasing a tight muscle.

The exact location and number of needles placed depend on the condition being treated. Usually no more than eight to ten needles are used per treatment. Once the needles are in place, several things may occur, depending on the practitioner and the nature of the pain. One possibility is—nothing. The needles are left untouched until they are removed. If additional stimulation is needed or desired, however, the acupuncturist may rotate the needles quickly or slowly in one direction or another. Others use electroacupuncture, in which an electric stimulator is attached to the needles to deliver a low-voltage electrical current. According to some practitioners, this technique greatly improves the effectiveness of the treatment.

## How Does Acupuncture Work?

Several theories have been suggested, as discussed in "Acupressure." For acupuncture in particular, the endorphin theory is supported by an increased level of endorphins found in the cerebrospinal fluid after acupuncture treatment.

Western science has yet to adequately measure or explain how acupuncture works, which leads some researchers to claim that it works because of the placebo effect. This means that because people believe it will work, it does. This claim, however, does not explain why acupuncture relieves pain in animals. Some researchers do agree, however, that the trigger points are the optimum sites for acupuncture and the basis for its success.

Acupuncture can provide dramatic relief for people with backache, including those with a herniated disk or sciatica. In fact acupuncture is the most commonly used treatment for sciatica in China. Many people report feeling euphoric for hours and even weeks after an acupuncture session. For individuals with chronic pain the greatest relief sometimes comes one or two days after the treatment. In most cases of back pain, referral to an osteopath is made by the acupuncturist so that the individual can begin to deal with any structural problems.

## ALEXANDER TECHNIQUE

The Alexander Technique is about mind-body awareness; it helps you replace dysfunctional movements you do every day with healthier ones. These are movements you do unconsciously—walking, combing your hair, reaching for a glass, or picking up a package. When these habits are done inefficiently, they build stress, muscle tension, and fatigue and can result in pain, poor posture, and inflexibility, among other complaints.

The main objective of the Alexander Technique is to "maintain the poise of the head on top of the lengthening spine in movement and at rest." This wisdom was set forth by F. Matthais Alexander, who developed the Alexander Technique. He realized that most people, including himself, have a habit of pressing the head back and down and compressing the spine. This posture creates tension and inhibits both flexibility and movement. When he stopped these habits and allowed his neck to be free, his head to go forward and up, and his spine and torso to lengthen, he experienced new vitality, increased flexibility, and release of tension.

Good posture is much more than standing up straight—it's about maintaining good positions while you move. The movements taught by Alexander Technique teachers—they refer to themselves as teachers, not therapists—are designed to train the muscles to maintain good posture during routine movements such as sitting, standing, and walking. Alexander movements are not strenuous. Their purpose is to increase awareness of posture and how the body feels when it is in alignment.

You can evaluate your posture to help you decide if the Alexander Technique is a treatment you want to pursue. (See Appendix A for help in finding a practitioner.) If it is, you will need to work with a certified Alexander teacher in order to learn the technique properly. There are more than 2,500 Alexander teachers worldwide.

To evaluate your posture, stand unclothed in front of a full-length mirror. Be as objective as possible. This is not the time to think about how you would look on the beach. Your ultimate goal is reduced pain, healthy posture, and graceful motion. Answer the following questions based on what you see in the mirror:

FRONT VIEW:
Does my head sit squarely on my shoulders?
Do I cock my head to one side?
Does my chin jut too far forward?
Does my neck extend out in front of my body?

Do I hunch up or shrug my shoulders?
Is one shoulder higher than the other?
Are my shoulders rounded forward?
Do I draw in my chest?
Do I stand rigidly with my chest up high?
Is one hip higher than the other?
Do my arms hang evenly at my sides?
SIDE VIEW:
Do I overarch my back?
Do I hold my buttocks in too tight?
Does my stomach form a little shelf?
Do I try to suck in my stomach?

## Out with the Old: Three Components

To modify old habits, the Alexander Technique teaches that people must have conscious control of their behavior. You can accomplish this via three essential components: Be aware of the habit, inhibit your reaction, and develop a new mental direction.

Melissa had an opportunity to learn how these components work during her first few sessions with her Alexander teacher. Melissa had been working full-time as a data-entry clerk for eighteen months when she first went to see an Alexander teacher. All of the clerks in Melissa's office had a special chair that offers excellent lower back support, yet even with the proper chair Melissa had experienced neck and upper back pain for the past year. Because Melissa had a very specific complaint, the Alexander teacher addressed that concern immediately. She asked Melissa to re-create her work space and show how she performed her job. Then she observed how Melissa drank coffee, ate soup, brushed her teeth, and drove her car. The outcome of this unusual session was that the teacher noticed what Melissa had not: that she unconsciously hunched her shoulders during these activities. This unconscious habit compressed her spine and placed stress and tension on Melissa's neck and upper back muscles.

Thus the first step was accomplished: Melissa was aware of the habit. Now she needed to inhibit it. This required her to consciously control her behavior in the split second between the stimulus and her response to it. To help herself inhibit her ingrained responses, Melissa taped the words "Until I give up my habits, I have no free choice" over her computer terminal and around her apartment. Her teacher emphasized that Melissa could not make her shoulders stay down. Rather she was to inhibit the response and let the new habit emerge as she continued her activity. *Let* and *allow* are key words to Alexander Technique students. If you make yourself relax, you create more tension.

She continued to take lessons once or twice a week for several months, then once every two weeks for a total of thirty-two lessons. Most teachers of the Alexander Technique suggest that students take as many lessons as they feel are helpful to them.

## What Should I Expect from an Alexander Technique Session?

Most Alexander teachers work one-on-one with their students in sessions that typically last thirty to sixty minutes each. Some teachers now offer group classes; however, you will not receive the individual attention you can get in private lessons. Alexander teachers do not follow rigid programs or systems: Each lesson is tailored to the needs of the student. You will not undergo a physical examination or need to disrobe. After you discuss why you are seeking help and information about your job or any activities that could contribute to your back pain, the teacher may explain how the technique works or demonstrate some of the movements to you as he or she explains them.

During the actual lessons teachers use their hands to guide students through every movement—bending, sitting, standing, lying down, lifting, and so on. Some movements are taught while you stand; others while you lie on a treatment table. If you have a specific activity you want to address—for example your job requires that you often reach up to overhead shelves—the teacher will also work on those movements with you.

The teacher's job is to help you inhibit your habitual responses to certain stimuli and then help you select new reactions to take. You won't go home from a lesson with a list of exercises to do: There aren't any. You will be asked, however, to increase your awareness of how you move now, just as Melissa did. The more conscious you are of your physical behavior, the more likely your subconscious and your muscles will be reprogrammed to remember when you aren't thinking about it. This takes time and practice. When you practice, keep the following tips in mind:

- If possible, do the movements in front of a full-length mirror so that you can monitor yourself. In the Alexander Technique careful adjustment of your spine and maintaining proper alignment are much more important than speed or repetition.
- Practice the movements every day. To get rid of old habits, you need to practice new ones daily.
- To help you keep your spine aligned, visualize that a long thread is being pulled from the top of your head, gently drawing your spine up straight, as if you were a puppet on a string.

# BIOFEEDBACK

*The real problem is not the pain, but how we handle it.*
*—Edward Abraham, M.D.*

Biofeedback is an excellent example of a technique that opens the door to a dialogue between you and your body. It allows you to have more control over your pain, to improve your concentration, and to achieve an overall feeling of relaxation.

Basically biofeedback involves the use of a device (at least initially) that measures what's going on physiologically with your body *(bio-)* and lets you know what that response is *(feedback)* via some kind of signal, such as beeps or blinking lights or a moving needle on a screen. The devices are typically electronic instruments that have electrodes, which are placed on the skin over muscles. The responses these electrodes pick up are transmitted to the biofeedback machine, which then provides you input on such body functions as heart rate, muscle tension, skin temperature, and blood pressure.

Barry had chronic lower back pain for which he took analgesics and intermittently followed a movement routine. He also claimed that he "concentrated on relaxing," but it didn't seem to help. A friend suggested biofeedback, which combines relaxation and imagery (see also "Visualization and Guided Imagery").

At the biofeedback clinic the therapist explained that she would measure the amount of muscle tension in Barry's back by placing electrodes on the lumbar area. After she placed the sensors, the therapist asked Barry to concentrate on relaxing his muscles and releasing the tension in his back. The machine provided instant feedback, via a beeping sound, which showed Barry he was not relaxing at all.

Barry was surprised: "But I'm trying so hard to relax,"

he said, which the therapist believed was the reason the pain persisted. Instead the therapist led Barry through a guided-imagery exercise and then suggested Barry continue with visualization to help decrease his tension. Visualization and biofeedback are a common combination that is very effective in treating back pain as well as many other conditions.

Barry focused on images of a hiking trip he had taken in South Dakota. He recalled the colorful sunsets, the smell of wildflowers, the sound of the wind whistling through the evergreens. After several sessions Barry significantly decreased the amount of muscle tension in his back by using these images, and monitored his progress with the biofeedback machine: The slower the beeps, the more his muscles relaxed. He had established a dialogue with his back pain, and his body responded. Once Barry knew which images worked for him and how his body could respond, he created the same relaxation at home without the biofeedback machine.

Biofeedback is mostly used for chronic rather than acute back pain, as it usually takes several weeks of training before people can achieve the control they need to significantly reduce pain. You will need to find a biofeedback clinic or center or a biofeedback therapist who has the equipment and expertise to help you (see Appendix A).

---

**HOW TO CHOOSE A BIOFEEDBACK THERAPIST**

- Talk to individuals who are licensed to practice independently or under the supervision of a licensed professional. Most biofeedback therapists are also psychologists; some are physicians, nurses, physical therapists, or other health care professionals.
- The Biofeedback Certification Institute of America issues

certificates to individuals who pass their high standards for training, experience, and education. Therapists without the certificate certainly may be as qualified as those with it.

- Ask therapists what kind of medical conditions they work with most often. If a therapist has little experience with back pain, you may want to find someone who does.
- Does the therapist answer all your questions patiently? Do you feel comfortable asking them, or are you made to feel ignorant? Your comfort is critical; the last thing you need is more stress. If you do not feel at ease, find another therapist.

Researchers report some mixed results on biofeedback; however, it has proven to be effective in individuals with severe pain and to make people feel they have greater control over their symptoms. If you are highly motivated, you will likely succeed. Complement the biofeedback with other forms of relaxation therapy such as breathing, visualization, or meditation.

## BREATHING THERAPY

Something as simple—and as vital—as breathing properly can help alleviate your back pain. Most of us don't think about how we are breathing unless our lungs are congested or we have a condition that makes breathing difficult. We're alive and kicking, so we must be breathing correctly— right? Wrong. Watch how babies breathe. They breathe from the diaphragm, which makes their belly rise and fall. This is the most natural and healthy way to breathe. As adults we have forgotten how to do this: We tend to take shallow chest breaths instead.

Deep, concentrated breathing practiced several times a day can revitalize your back and make you feel good all over because it releases stress and tension. You can practice breathing therapy in your office, while you watch television, when you sit in traffic—any place and time that is comfortable for you. The following approaches are suggestions.

## Breathing for Pain Relief

Several different deep-breathing methods can help bring your entire body into balance, reduce back pain, and allow your energy to flow freely. The first few times you practice breathing techniques you may want to pick a quiet spot where you won't be interrupted for several minutes. Once you know how proper breathing feels, you can do it anywhere.

Lie down on your back with your knees bent, or sit in a comfortable chair, and loosen any tight clothing. Place your hands over your abdomen and rib cage so that you can feel how they move as you breathe. First, try the most basic method—*deep breathing*. Take a deep breath and send that breath deep into your abdomen. Feel your belly rise, and then as the breath moves up into your diaphragm and upper lungs, they, too, will expand. Hold that breath for a few seconds, then slowly release it. Repeat this cycle several times slowly, and each time concentrate on your breath and the rise and fall of your abdomen, diaphragm, and lungs.

Another breathing technique is called *hara breathing*. Take one hand and place it on a spot three fingers width below your navel. This is an acupressure point called Conception Vessel 6, also known as the *hara,* or "the sea of energy." Concentrate on this spot as you breathe deeply into your belly. Feel your lower abdomen rise and fall as you slowly breathe in and out. This concentrated breathing method helps strengthen the lower back.

Some people find that visualizing their breath as a healing substance helps relieve pain (see "Visualization and Guided Imagery"). Once you are comfortable, close your eyes (if you choose) and concentrate on the area that is painful. As you take a deep breath, send the breath to that area. Imagine that your breath is releasing your tight muscles or easing the tension in that spot. Hold that breath for several seconds and then release it slowly. Visualize your pain leaving with your exhaled breath. Repeat this cycle slowly and comfortably; take five to ten minutes if you can.

You may want to try an exercise in which you concentrate only on your breathing. You or a friend can make a cassette tape of the brief example below so that you can use it again and again. (Commercial tapes also are available; see Appendix B.) If you record it, speak slowly and clearly. Feel free to modify the script: it is a guideline only. Allow five to ten minutes for the exercise, and choose a time and place you will not be disturbed.

Breathe in slowly through your nose to a count of seven. Hold the breath for a second or two. As you breathe out, let your lips relax, slightly parted. Release the breath slowly and easily. Feel your belly fall, your back relax. Feel the calm that comes with release of your breath.

Breathe in and feel your belly expand and rise. Feel your breath move slowly and easily into your chest. Your chest expands like a balloon and then gently releases its air. Feel your breath leave through your parted lips. As the breath leaves, feel it take tension from your back. See yourself becoming more relaxed. As you inhale again, breathe in relaxation. Send the breath to your pain and relax the muscles as you breathe in. As you breathe out, feel the tension go with the breath.

Every inhale gently stretches the ligaments around

your spine. As you breathe in, the spaces between your vertebrae open up and tension is released from your ligaments. Every in-breath cleanses and releases. Every out-breath cleanses and releases. The very act of deep breathing reduces your pain.

As you breathe in and out, focus on the hara, the spot that is three finger widths below your navel. Breathe into this spot and feel it grow warm. As you breathe in, imagine that the hara opens up and allows your back pain in. As you exhale, see your back pain ride that breath up through your belly, your diaphragm, your lungs. See it leave through your parted lips. As you breathe out, see the tension leave your body.

As you breathe in, feel the warmth radiate from your hara. Feel it spread to your pelvis and to your hips. As you exhale, feel any tension leave with that breath. Feel the warmth ride with your breath as it leaves your belly, your diaphragm, and your upper chest. With every in-breath feel the warmth spread into your buttocks and down into your legs and feet. Feel as the breath releases the tension.

Every time you inhale, feel your lower spine open and relax. Feel your midtorso gently expand as you breathe in. As you move the breath out, feel relaxation move in as your entire midtorso gently relaxes toward your spine.

Feel your chest walls expand and stretch as you inhale. The spine of your upper back arches gently as you breathe in. As you release your breath, let go of any tension. Feel the stress leave your chest and your back.

Feel each breath as it enters your throat. Every in-breath causes your chin to tilt up slightly as your upper chest moves. As you release your breath, your chin settles down slightly. Feel your neck open up to the in-breath; feel your neck settle back when the breath is released. Take a deep breath and feel your shoulders lift up and out slightly. Feel your neck muscles relax. Release the air slowly from your belly, diaphragm, and upper chest. The out-breath releases the shoulder girdle to its most comfortable position.

End your breathing session by taking a complete, slow, deep unifying breath. Feel the breath throughout your body and your mind. Allow the breath to penetrate every corner of your being. Hold it for several seconds and then release it slowly. Release all tension. Allow in peace and calm.

Deep-breathing techniques are at the center of many Eastern disciplines and general health practices. We suggest you make deep breathing part of your daily routine.

## CHIROPRACTIC

Chiropractic is the largest drug-free health care profession in the United States. Some people in the conventional medicine arena say it's an unscientific practice and that its practitioners are quacks. Yet more than 15 million people a year visit chiropractors. Most of the individuals who go to a chiropractor do so for musculoskeletal problems, such as lower back pain, whiplash injuries, sciatica, neck pain, and disk problems.

Many reports support the use of chiropractic. According to the results of a large study of the use of manipulation for lower back pain, chiropractic is effective in individuals with acute or subacute lower back pain either with or without evidence of neurological involvement or sciatic nerve irritation. A comparison study of chiropractic and hospital outpatient treatment found chiropractic slightly better for people with chronic or severe low back pain, and this advantage was still apparent after two years.

Central to chiropractic is the idea that the true cause of disease is within the body and makes individuals susceptible to external factors such as viruses, cancer-causing chemicals, and other environmental factors. Chiropractic is based on the following concepts:

- The vertebrae frequently become misaligned and cause interference of nerve signals from the brain to the organs and tissues. The name for misalignments of vertebrae is *subluxation*. They may or may not show up on an X ray.
- Manipulation of the spine restores alignment of the vertebrae, which in turn frees the body of nerve interference. This adjustment helps reduce or eliminate the body's susceptibility to outside forces and allows it to function properly and heal itself.

Chiropractic adjustment and osteopathic manipulation are similar in that both return the vertebrae and joints to a normal or more functional state so that the body can heal itself. Generally chiropractors feel for displaced vertebrae rather than decreased function and mobility. Once they locate the problem area, they apply pressure to the bone itself and use force to correct the misalignment. Osteopaths, in contrast, look for impaired mobility and function and use manipulation to correct dysfunctional muscles by applying minimal force or thrust. Another basic difference is that because chiropractors are not licensed physicians, the scope of their practice is more limited than that of osteopaths and medical doctors (e.g., they cannot prescribe medications or perform surgery).

## Chiropractic for Your Back Pain

If you have never been to a chiropractor, you may be a bit nervous. (For help in finding a chiropractor, see Appendix A.)

---

### EVALUATING A CHIROPRACTOR

According to the ACA, evaluate a chiropractor (D.C.) for the following. Does he or she:

- Seem to be concerned about you as an individual?
- Have a clean, neat office?
- Provide emergency care?
- Provide another chiropractor to take calls if he/she is away?
- Explain the necessity for all exams and therapy and justify the need for treatment?
- Tell you about the treatment before doing it and get your permission to do it?
- Explain how many visits may be necessary? (If treatment is going to help, you should feel better within four to six weeks.) Remember, most chiropractors are not medical doctors, therefore they are not licensed to perform surgery or prescribe medications. Some, however, are both M.D.s and D.C.s.

---

Leonard had those same thoughts, but the fact that he had recurring lower back pain that was interfering with his job as a carpenter motivated him to shelve his apprehensions. Before being ushered into an examination room, Leonard filled out a case-history form. In addition to the questions found on routine medical forms, this one asked specifically about any past accidents, broken bones, falls, sprains, or concussions, as well as whether his birth had been cesarean.

When Leonard met the chiropractor, she immediately asked him to talk about his symptoms, the events surrounding the time his back pain started, what kind of work he did, and what other activities he was involved in. She then showed him a model of the spine and several back and muscle diagrams and explained how the muscles, vertebrae, and ligaments were interconnected. Only then did she begin the physical and neurologic examination.

Leonard's chiropractor used a sensing instrument called a *surface electromyograph (EMG),* which measures the amount of electrical current in the spinal muscles. Electrodes from the EMG were attached to several locations near Leonard's spine as he performed various movements, such as sitting, lifting each knee toward his chest, tilting his head to either side, and lifting his arms. The EMG indicates where spinal subluxations occur.

After detaching the electrodes, the chiropractor asked Leonard to lean into the adjustable padded table so that she could examine his back. A chiropractic treatment table (see Figure II-5) can be moved into a vertical position so that people with back pain do not have to climb onto a fixed-height table. It also has openings and adjustments that allow the chiropractor to make the patient as comfortable as possible.

While Leonard lay on his stomach, the chiropractor began to palpate (examine by touch) down the entire length of his spine, feeling for any tender spots, inflammation, or bumps. Using a handheld device called a *thermeter,* she measured the skin temperature on either side of Leonard's spine. A lower temperature on one side versus the other indicates possible nerve interference. To help rule out the possibility of a physical condition, most chiropractors will also take a spinal X ray. Beyond that, however, be cautious

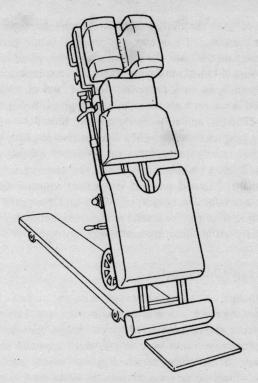

**II-5  Chiropractic treatment table**

of any chiropractor who wants to prescribe expensive tests, as they are rarely justified.

Now Leonard was ready for his first treatment. Chiropractic treatments are typically called *adjustments,* and usually are done with the palms. Not all chiropractors do adjustments in the same way, however. Some have a gentle approach, whereas others use sudden, thrusting maneuvers to realign the bones. The kind of treatment you receive will depend on the type of training your chiropractor received, the condition of your back, and the results of your X rays.

Leonard soon discovered that his chiropractor used both approaches, which is a common practice. While Leonard was lying on the table, the chiropractor gently lifted his leg up toward his chest. She then placed her knee on his upper thigh, one hand on his opposite shoulder, and then swiftly pressed down on both. The "crack" Leonard heard came from his back, and surprisingly it didn't hurt.

The next ten minutes were a combination of gentle pressure and more rapid adjustments. When it was all over, Leonard felt a bit achy but no pain. The chiropractor suggested that Leonard schedule subsequent adjustments one week apart for the next three weeks and also gave him written instructions for several movement routines designed to strengthen his back and abdominal muscles.

## Types of Chiropractic

Although no two backaches are alike and no two chiropractors approach a case in the same exact way, Leonard's experience can be considered typical. When you choose a chiropractor, you may want to ask which approach she or he uses. Some chiropractors diagnose based solely on touch; others never proceed with an adjustment without taking X rays. Your chiropractor may use a handheld instrument called an Activator, which is a small rubber-tipped tool used to gently and painlessly move the vertebrae.

Basically there are three kinds of chiropractors. Some adhere to the "Law of the Nerve," which means they treat all disease using manipulation. Such practitioners are called *straights,* and many in the chiropractic profession are moving away from this thought. Most chiropractors are considered *mixers.* These chiropractors take a more holistic approach and integrate other therapies into their work, such as acupuncture, diet, massage, and thermotherapy; and they do not claim to be able to treat all disease. A third group are known as *network chiropractors*. Their approach is to combine various chiropractic techniques, which allows them to adjust subluxations with the precise amount and type of force suggested by X rays and other clinical findings.

## How Does Chiropractic Work?

Chiropractic is based on the concept that different parts of the spine are connected to specific areas of the nervous system. To reduce or eliminate pain, chiropractors manipulate the joints and the area of the spine that corresponds to the location of the pain, thus relieving pressure or tension on the nerves and vertebrae.

The number of treatments you need will depend on many factors, including the severity and cause of the back pain, your overall strength and flexibility, and which other therapies you are pursuing. One treatment is rarely enough to correct the problem. If you have good strength in your back but suffer from back strain or tension that is continuously aggravated by your occupation, for example, you may need only two or three treatments followed by periodic readjustments every three to six months. In contrast a case of sciatica may require twelve to fifteen treatments followed by a checkup every three months. You and your chiropractor can work out a schedule that fits your needs.

# CRANIOSACRAL THERAPY

To a craniosacral therapist the indicator of a person's health and well-being is the cerebrospinal fluid—the colorless substance that protects the brain and spinal cord from physical injury. Craniosacral therapy is a type of osteopathic manipulation in which practitioners relieve tension in the head by making subtle manipulations to the skull, sacrum (lower back), or other parts of the body. This therapy requires highly developed palpatory skills (a very keen sense of touch). Very few osteopaths practice this therapy; in fact most craniosacral practitioners are physical therapists, massage therapists, and other bodywork professionals.

## Craniosacral Therapy for Your Back Pain

Craniosacral therapy is a highly specialized skill and requires a licensed craniosacral therapist or professional osteopath who has been trained in the technique. See Appendix A for information on how to find the appropriate practitioner.

After conducting a physical examination and obtaining a medical and personal history, a typical session with a craniosacral therapist may involve the following. You will lie on your back on a padded treatment table, and the therapist will gently and very lightly grasp your head from behind. The bones that make up the skull move with an inward-outward or forward-backward motion. When the bones do not move in sync, the practitioner can usually feel a pulling motion. He or she can either "ride" this pull to its extreme, hold it there and follow it as it returns to a normal rhythm, or directly guide the imbalanced motion back to normal using a very subtle, yet very powerful pull with the hands. Whenever the therapist applies pressure, seldom does it exceed the equivalent weight of a nickel.

There are three basic approaches to craniosacral therapy: sutural, meningeal, and reflex. Therapists who practice the *sutural* method manipulate the sutures of the skull—where the bones meet—in order to relieve pressure (see Figure II-6). In the *meningeal* approach the practitioner manipulates the meninges, which releases any restrictions of the cranial sutures and the underlying membranes. The *reflex* approach relieves stress in the craniosacral system as well as other structures and organs by stimulating the nerve endings in the scalp or between the sutures. A fourth approach, called the Sacro-Occipital Technique, is a combination of the three methods. Regardless of the approach used, many people report feeling an incredible sense of peace and calm during treatment, so much so that they drift off into a hypnotic state or fall asleep.

## How Does Craniosacral Therapy Work?

As the cerebrospinal fluid bathes the central nervous system, it creates an undulating rhythm called the *central respiratory movement*. As the ventricles of the brain pulse with the release of the cerebrospinal fluid, the bones of the skull expand and contract. Craniosacral therapists, who ad-

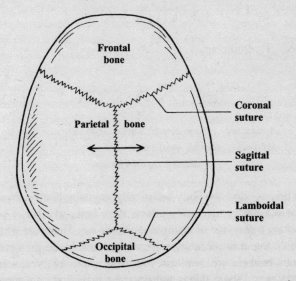

**II-6  Bones and sutures of the skull**

mit that this movement is minute, monitor this motion by feeling with their hands or watching a person's subtle body movements and determining where the flow is blocked. Once the blockage is located, the practitioner makes slight adjustments in the head or spine and releases the pressure.

How do blockages occur? Craniosacral therapists believe that all the bumps, blows, and bruises the head receives from the moment it makes its appearance outside the birth canal cause the bones in the head to shift or jam up. These bones are held together by connective tissue called sutures, which allow craniosacral practitioners to manipulate the bones, realign them, free up and rebalance the flow of fluid, and stretch the membranes in the head. For individuals with back pain the result is often pain relief and greater mobility.

# CRYOTHERAPY

See "Hydrotherapy."

# DIET/NUTRITION

*A man may esteem himself happy when that which is his food is also his medicine.*
—*Henry David Thoreau*

When we view the body holistically, anything that we do to the outside or the inside affects the whole, whether it be getting a massage or eating a chocolate bar. Therefore what you eat and drink have an impact on your blood pressure, body temperature, how fast your nails grow, and, yes, your back pain. Some things influence the body and pain more directly than others. We will look at a few of them below.

## Weight

Back pain strikes people who are under-, over-, and of average weight, yet there is evidence that excess weight is a risk for back pain, especially if it is in the abdomen. Excess baggage in the stomach area pulls the spine forward in the spot where most back pain occurs: the five vertebrae of the lower back (lumbar) region. These vertebrae are the most vulnerable to stress because they are supported only by the abdominal muscles. Weak abdominal muscles are a big contributing factor in back pain. When the muscles lack strength and tone and there is excess weight in the same area, the combination can spell double trouble for your back. To compensate for the excess weight, the back muscles increase their tension, which increases the pressure on the lower back. For example, for every extra pound in the abdominal area, up to five pounds of pressure are placed on the back. If you are carrying ten extra pounds in the abdomen, the increased strain on your lower back is fifty pounds.

## Diet and Your Back Pain

Many holistic practitioners address the importance of a sound nutritional program. Typically their recommendations include a plan that contains lots of whole grains and cereals, vegetables, fruits, beans and legumes, and nuts, little or no dairy products, and no meat or fish. Alcohol, caffeine, and sugars are best avoided as well. Some practitioners recommend a macrobiotic diet—a rigid style that some people find hard to adopt at first.

Any modifications you make to your diet should be done gradually and steadily to allow time for your body to adjust. If you never or rarely eat beans or legumes (an excellent protein source without the fat and cholesterol present in meat), for example, and suddenly eat several servings a day, you may experience gas and indigestion. Likewise, dropping dairy and meat products from your diet will likely result in lower cholesterol levels, a drop in weight, higher energy levels, as well as a lower risk of heart disease, diabetes, stroke, some forms of cancer, and many other ailments.

Your perspective of yourself and your pain are also key to making dietary modifications. When a health practitioner says, "Modify your diet," some people immediately think, "Look what I have to give up!" Instead an approach such as "Look at all the things I never thought about eating before. What an adventure!" is a much healthier and more positive attitude.

Vivian, a fifty-six-year-old secretary who suffered from chronic lower back pain for more than three years, turned on to biofeedback and turned off the animal products in her diet. Six months later her pain is under control, her energy level is higher than its been in years ("I feel twenty-five again"), and she shed twelve pounds without dieting. "At first I thought I would miss certain foods, such as ice cream. But I found wonderful substitutes that taste good, and so many other new foods I had never tried before. It's been a real exciting experience for me."

Modifications to diet and the addition of nutritional supplements are preventive and maintenance approaches to back-pain control, and will contribute to your overall treatment program to reduce or eliminate your back pain.

## Vitamins and Supplements

A conscientious supplement program, along with a healthful eating plan, can help keep your muscles, bones, ligaments, and other tissues healthy and strong and help prevent and reduce pain or prevent recurring episodes.

Most physicians who recommend supplement programs

for back pain generally agree on which supplements are beneficial; they do not always agree on how much of each supplement people should take. We pooled the research and have given you some suggested supplements and a dosage range for each. Consult with your practitioner for your specific needs.

- *Boron:* 3 mg (milligrams) daily; improves calcium uptake. Discontinue this supplement once the pain is healed, unless you are age fifty or older. The human requirement for boron has not been established and long-term toxicity studies have not been completed.
- *Bromelain:* 1,000–1,400 mg per day, divided into three doses. This enzyme, derived from pineapple, relieves muscle tension and prevents blood clots. It is not known to cause adverse effects.
- *Calcium/Magnesium:* in a 2:1 ratio, at bedtime, 1,500–2,000 mg of calcium and 700–1,000 mg of magnesium (chelated form). The National Institutes of Health recommend not exceeding 2,000 mg of calcium per day, as it can interfere with absorption of iron and zinc and may cause kidney stones in susceptible individuals.
- *Dl-Phenylalanine:* an essential amino acid that acts as an analgesic that is better than aspirin for pain. It increases the level of release of endogenous endorphin-like substances and helps reduce inflammation. Take 250 mg fifteen to thirty minutes before meals. If pain is not relieved within three weeks, double the dosage for another three weeks. Do not use if you are pregnant, hypertensive, diabetic, or have phenylketonuria (an inability to oxidize phenylalanine).
- *Fish oil supplement (cholesterol-free), such as Max-EPA:* 1,000 mg three times daily for back pain associated with arthritis. Not much is known about long-term

side effects. Avoid cod liver oil as a source of fish oil, as it contains excessive vitamin A.

- *Vitamin B complex:* 25–50 mg twice daily. The B vitamins are water soluble (easily eliminated from the body), and toxicity is extremely rare.
- *Vitamin B1:* 1,000–4,000 mg daily (only under medical supervision) along with B12 injections (see below).
- *Vitamin B12:* 5,000–10,000 IU daily by injection (by your physician).
- *Vitamin C:* 1,500–10,000 mg per day with meals. May cause stomach discomfort or diarrhea at 5,000 mg or more daily. Reducing the dose eliminates these problems.
- *Vitamin E:* 400 IU once or twice daily. More than 1,000 IU daily promotes clotting and suppresses immunity.
- *Zinc:* 50 mg daily. More than 100 mg daily can suppress immunity.

In addition to these supplements, some naturopaths suggest a potassium chloride and iron phosphate combination for pain caused by inflammation, such as occurs with a herniated disk.

---

### A GOOD DAILY VITAMIN/MINERAL PROGRAM

Doctors frequently disagree as to what constitutes optimal dosages of any vitamin or mineral needed for good health. Many people follow the RDA (Recommended Daily Allowance) as stated by the FDA, but those levels were set to prevent the development of serious disease, not ensure a vital, healthy lifestyle. To do that, you need to consume a balanced variety of healthy foods and follow a supplement program that works for your needs.

According to Dr. Robert M. Giller, author of *Natural Prescriptions,* a good, general supplement that has at least 50 mg each of vitamins B1, B2, and B6 usually also has a good balance of the other vitamins, minerals, and trace minerals the body needs. If you cannot find a supplement with these levels, you will need to take more than one supplement. In addition to the levels of B vitamins mentioned above, he recommends that your daily general supplement(s) contain the following levels of these antioxidants:

1,000 mg vitamin C
400–600 IU vitamin E
100–200 mcg selenium

These are considered to be minimum maintenance levels. The dosages of vitamin C, calcium, and vitamin E mentioned in the text for back pain are in addition to this daily recommended amount.

## Foods to Enjoy and Foods to Avoid

There are dozens of sound nutritional choices for you to explore, everything from kamut to kiwi; from amaranth to zucchini. But, you argue, you like steak and hot dogs and ice cream, yet we're suggesting you eliminate them. What do they have to do with back pain?

Meat and dairy products are more than harbors of fat, cholesterol, calories, and contaminants. Excess calcium in the diet can cause spurs (bony growths) to form. When you eliminate meat and milk products from the diet, the calcium mechanism in the body can readjust and help avoid this painful condition. Too much fat in the diet disturbs the flow of energy in the body, including the meninges and spinal column. This leads to mechanical complications in the spine. Red meat, as well as fowl and fish, also cause muscles to swell, shorten, and become sluggish and stiff, particularly in the mid and lower back. Animal protein products, such as meat and dairy, for example, contain uric acid, which builds up in the joints and causes inflammation and pain.

The teaspoonful of white sugar you put into your coffee and on your cereal and the sugar hidden in many foods and beverages are all taking a toll on your back. When sugar is metabolized, it places a strain on the adrenal glands, which are located on top of the kidneys. But what does this have to do with back pain?

According to Chinese medicine, pain and tension in the lower back are associated with the kidneys, the bladder, and the reproductive system. If your kidneys are under stress—from overworked adrenal glands, from eating too much salt, drinking too much or not enough liquid, or from an excess of fear or sexual activity, for example—you may feel pain in your lower back. When blood sugar levels rise, they put stress on the pancreas, kidneys, and spleen, which places additional strain on the lower back.

Health professionals from the East have some definite ideas about which foods help back pain. They include the following:

- *Star Anise:* Fry this herb and grind it into a powder. Dissolve 1¼ tsp. of the powder with a little salt in a cup of warm water. Take this twice a day to cure low back pain.
- *Hawthorn Fruit:* Prepare a hawthorn wine by combining 1 cup hawthorn slices, 1 cup fresh longans, 1 oz. red dates, 2 tbsp. brown sugar, and 4½ cups rice wine. Allow this mixture to marinate for ten days. (Hawthorn fruit slices are available in most Chinese herb

shops or by mail order.) Drink 1 to 2 oz. of hawthorn fruit wine at bedtime to relieve lumbago and muscle pain.

- *Walnuts:* Boil 1 tbsp. walnuts with 1 tbsp. crushed fresh ginger. Drink this mixture twice a day to relieve pain.

# FELDENKRAIS METHOD

Dr. Moshe Feldenkrais believed people learn just enough physical movement to function and then leave most of their potential undeveloped and unexplored. A simple example can demonstrate this. Clasp your hands together, folded as if in prayer. Is your right thumb over your left or your left over your right? Clasp your hands again, but this time consciously switch which thumb is on top. Does it feel strange? The way you always clasp your hands is a habit and one you can change if you want to. It is simply a matter of awareness and reeducation.

## Feldenkrais and Your Back Pain

Like practitioners of the Alexander Technique (see page 82), those trained in the Feldenkrais Method emphasize that they are teachers and you are the student. Their purpose is to teach you to move your body to program your brain and allow it to reach its potential. To accomplish this, the Feldenkrais Method consists of more than a thousand different movements. Feldenkrais practitioners use a combination of these movements along with one-on-one manipulation to gradually reeducate the body to function more efficiently. This approach is very successful in treating chronic back pain, relieving muscle tension, improving posture, and increasing flexibility.

All Feldenkrais movements are done while you are fully clothed in loose, comfortable attire. You will do many of the movements on a padded table or on the floor, where your teacher will slowly and gently guide you into positions that are without strain or pain. Each movement is designed to increase your awareness of your body and the communication between it and your mind. Lessons typically last thirty to seventy-five minutes, and the number of lessons you need will depend on the extent of your pain and your physical condition. Generally it is recommended that you begin with two lessons a week. To locate a Feldenkrais teacher in your area, see Appendix A.

## FOLD AND HOLD

The body is smart: It has a natural tendency to move into a comfortable position, especially when there is a painful or tender spot. Children do this; they often sleep in what we might consider to be a twisted or uncomfortable position, yet their body has "found" the position naturally.

Fold and Hold is the brainchild of an orthopedic surgeon, Dr. Dale L. Anderson, who studied how the body moves naturally to relieve pain, as well as the effectiveness of "man-made" methods. After researching and experimenting with these and other osteopathic techniques, Dr. Anderson developed Fold and Hold, a pain-relief technique that builds on nature's wisdom. He estimates that 75 percent of common aches and pains are reduced or eliminated using this method. The remaining 25 percent are caused by inflammation, infections, tumors, and various forms of trauma—causes that Fold and Hold is not designed to handle.

Fold and Hold is composed of four basic steps:

1. Identify a painful area.
2. Fold your body over the painful spot until you find a position in which the pain is completely or about 75 percent improved.
3. Hold that comfortable position for at least ninety seconds.
4. Return slowly to a normal position.

All movements in Fold and Hold are done slowly, gently, and always with comfort as the goal. You don't need any equipment, and you can do the movements just about anywhere. Fold and Hold works by relieving muscle spasm, one of the chief causes of back pain, by relaxing and stretching the affected muscles. The result is pain relief, and if there are other factors involved in the pain, such as swelling or tissue damage, release from the spasm allows you to address them now in a more relaxed way. If you experience more pain, stop. If you don't experience improvement with Fold and Hold after three sessions, or if the pain gets worse, see your doctor. Your pain may be caused by something other than muscle spasm.

For maximum pain relief, use Fold and Hold in conjunction with other therapies. Reflexology, heat, massage, ice, and other natural therapies complement Fold and Hold.

Following are three Fold and Hold techniques for the lower back.

## Fold and Hold A

This position helps pain brought on by sitting in a slouched or hunched-over position, say at a computer terminal or your desk. You may feel a nagging lower back pain that improves when you bend forward and worsens when you stand or walk. For this Fold and Hold, Dr. Anderson often suggests people hold the position for up to ten minutes.

- Sit on the floor or anywhere you can sit comfortably and safely curled up into a ball—bring your knees up to your chest, chin, or ears, whichever is most comfortable (see Figure II-7).
- Strive for comfort. If that means you need to squirm or twist a little, do it. Listen to what your body is saying to you.
- Hold the position for ninety seconds or longer and then slowly return to your normal position.

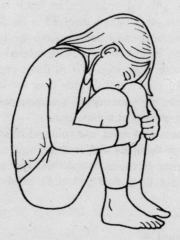

**II-7   Fold and Hold for low back and abdominal pain**

## Fold and Hold B

If you have low back pain that improves when you stand or walk, you may feel one or more tender spots on the back side of your vertebrae. This is where the muscles that bridge the vertebrae are located. This type of back pain can be caused by repetitive lifting or by any motion that causes the back muscles to lengthen rapidly and go into spasm. To relieve this type of pain, try one or both of the following Fold and Hold techniques.

- Stand with your back to a table or other piece of sturdy furniture, such as a sofa.
- Fold over the pain by arching your back backward (see Figure II-8). You may need to twist away or toward the tender spot a little until the pain subsides.
- An alternative fold is to lie on your stomach and prop yourself up on your elbows or hands, arching your back.

## Fold and Hold C

Runners, joggers, and power walkers often experience low back pain, pain in the buttocks, and sciatica. If you fall into this category, you may feel a very tender spot in a muscle in the midbuttock, called the *piriformis muscle*. This muscle allows you to rotate your leg outward. When the piriformis is in spasm, it presses against the sciatic nerve, which is under this muscle, and you feel pain, numbness, or both, in the leg.

- Locate the tender spot, which is usually in the middle of the buttock.
- Reduce the pain using one or more of the following Fold and Hold techniques:

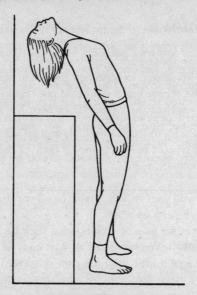

**II-8   Fold and Hold for low back and abdominal pain**

—While standing, put your foot up on a stool or drape your leg over the arm of a chair.

—Lie on your stomach and bring your affected leg up toward your head by bending your knee. This is sometimes called the frog position.

—Sit on a chair or sofa and bring your foot up to rest in front of you as if you were going to hug your knee. Then let your leg and knee fall comfortably out to the side.

After you do Fold and Hold C, you need to stretch the piriformis muscle. Do this by getting on your hands and knees. Lean back, keeping one leg stationary and letting the other extend out. Rest your buttocks on the heel of the foot just behind you. If the pain is on the right side, bring your left leg over the right leg and move your left buttock toward your right foot. Reverse the movement if the pain is on the left side. This movement stretches the piriformis muscle.

Sometimes the tender spot isn't where you think it should be. Madelaine experienced pain that caused her to walk stooped forward, and she could not stand up straight. When she searched for a tender spot near her lower right side, where the pain was located, she could not find it. That's because the tender spot for such back pain is often lurking in the abdominal muscles, groin, or pubic area. Once Madelaine found the tender spot in her abdominal area, she did Fold and Hold A, above, three times a day for a week, and felt significant relief after the first day.

## Beyond Fold and Hold

While Fold and Hold techniques are a pain treatment, prevention is usually on the minds of back-pain sufferers. Dr. Anderson emphasizes that there are other strategies to use in conjunction with Fold and Hold that help prevent recurrence of back pain. These include (1) stretching the muscle that you treat with Fold and Hold, as well as the connective tissue that surrounds the muscle; (2) doing movements to strengthen weak muscles; (3) being conscious of and maintaining good posture in everything you do; (4) learning to distinguish between "good" and "bad" pain; and (5) healing the emotional side of your pain.

For strategies 1 and 2 you can use techniques discussed elsewhere in this section, especially under "Movement Therapy." Chapter 3 will help you with strategy 3, as will the Alexander Technique and the Feldenkrais Method.

For strategy 4: Some pain is good, even necessary, for healing to occur. Think of good pain as being discomfort. Perhaps you played several sets of tennis in the morning and when you got up from your chair after lunch, your legs ached. Good pain. Or you start your evening jog and your hamstrings hurt and feel tight so you stop and stretch. Good pain. Generally pain that occurs at the beginning of an activity and then lessens or disappears is good pain (discomfort). Pain that grows worse as you continue with the activity and that may cause other symptoms, such as swelling or shooting pain, is probably bad. Once you recognize your own personal tolerance level for pain—and that pain is in the brain—you can learn when it is okay to keep moving and healing with minimal discomfort.

This brings us to strategy 5, which involves the mind-body connection, as discussed in Chapter 4. The influence of emotions and feelings on the body and vice versa cannot be denied. When you heal the emotional side of your back pain—for example, you recognize and deal with tensions that may be contributing to it or talk about how having chronic back pain makes you feel as a person—you uncover inner strength and are in more control of your pain. You may want to review Chapter 4 again to reinforce your personal mind-body connection.

## GRAVITY INVERSION

See "Traction."

## HELLERWORK

Hellerwork is a special integration of deep massage, movement education, and dialogue with a Hellerwork practitioner that is designed to help people learn how their movements and emotions affect the body and any pain they may have. Some who have participated in the Hellerwork program series have referred to it as a whole mind-body-spiritual experience.

After extensive study of Rolfing and Aston-Patterning (two bodywork therapies not discussed in this book; see "Suggestions for Further Reading" for more information), Joseph Heller, a professional engineer, developed his own theories about massage and movement. In the process he realized that the mind—emotions and attitudes—also plays an essential part in physical health and how we move. When he brought these three elements together, Hellerwork was born in 1978. Today there are more than three hundred trained Hellerwork practitioners in the United States.

## Hellerwork and Your Back Pain

The Hellerwork program offers healing benefits to people with various ailments, including back pain, headache, and depression. Each one-on-one Hellerwork session lasts ninety minutes and focuses on a different part of the body. The eleven sessions must be completed in sequence. The suggested frequency is one session a week, although people choose their own schedule.

Heller explains that the massage portion of the program "manipulates the connective tissue . . . to reduce tension and help realign the parts." The goal is to align the body with gravity, which he sees as more than just standing on the earth but as a recognition that we are one with the earth. To track movement and posture changes throughout the program, Hellerwork practitioners take "before" and "after" photographs of participants as they stand in front of a grid with a plumb line marking their posture. After each session, people can see their progress by comparing the photographs.

Here is a brief summary of the eleven sessions that make up Hellerwork. Each session is named by its theme.

*Session 1: Inspiration*
Focus: the rib cage and the muscles attached to it; how to open up your breathing and align the rib cage over the pelvis.

*Session 2: Standing on Your Own Feet*
Focus: the leg muscles and their alignment, with emphasis on self-support and sufficiency.

*Session 3: Reaching Out*
Focus: the arms, shoulders, and the side muscles; how to release tension in these areas and achieve vertical alignment to the sides of the torso. The session covers giving and receiving, assertion and aggression.

*Session 4: Control and Surrender*
Focus: release of tension and emotions held deep inside—including your inner torso from the shoulders to the pelvic floor and your inner thigh muscles.

*Session 5: The Guts*
Focus: the abdominal muscles and your gut feelings.

*Session 6: Holding Back*
Focus: the back muscles and spine and the tensions you hold there.

*Session 7: Losing Your Head*
Focus: the mind-body connection, with emphasis on the muscles of your face, neck, and head and how to release muscle tension and help align your head over your torso.

*Session 8: The Feminine*
Focus: the entire lower half of the body including the feet, pelvis, and legs. Not just for women!

*Session 9: The Masculine*
Focus: the entire upper half of the body, including the shoulders, rib cage, neck, and arms, with emphasis on how we express masculine energy. Not just for men!

*Session 10: Integration*
Focus: the major joints, including spine, knees, hips, shoulders, ankles, elbows, and wrists. This session emphasizes the integrity in your body.

*Session 11: Coming Out*
Focus: bringing it all together so that you can take what you've learned and make it part of your every moment.

## How Does Hellerwork Work?

Every Hellerwork session includes the three elements Heller believes are crucial for healing: massage, movement education, and dialogue. Heller believes dialogue is a critical part of Hellerwork because when people verbalize what's going on in their life and what's happening in their body, they can make the mind-body connection. This realization can change their attitude about their body, which ultimately affects its structure. According to Heller, how people hold themselves reflects what's going on inside. If a person's shoulders round forward in a position suggesting sadness and rejection and a therapist works with the individual to strengthen the muscles and improve posture, the person will eventually return to the rounded position if the reason for the sadness is not addressed and resolved. Thus Hellerwork is a holistic healing method.

## HERBAL MEDICINE

People have used herbs to heal the body and the mind since ancient times. Practitioners of herbal medicine have alternately been honored and murdered and the practice banned and celebrated. Today the resurgent interest in and use of herbs opens the doors to new—yet definitely not new— avenues of healing for people with various ailments and conditions, including back pain.

The healing power of herbs can offer backache sufferers relief from pain and stress as well as the insomnia that often accompanies the pain. Herbs help restore the body to its natural state of balance and act as a complement to other healing therapies. A tea (see "Herbal Recipes" in box, page 124) made of Prince's pine, valerian, lobelia, gingerroot, and marshmallow root, for example, is often used for muscle spasms, but it does not "cure" the spasm. It does, however, provide physical and emotional relief and allow the individual to better perform the movements that will strength and support the affected area.

---

### GUIDELINES FOR HERBAL USE

• Many people successfully treat themselves with herbal remedies for back pain and related symptoms. As with any substance, however, misuse may cause adverse effects. When used in their proper dosages, herbal remedies are safe, effective, and relatively inexpensive. Before using any herbal remedy, you should consult a knowledgeable herbalist, naturopath, or homeopath to help you select the botanicals that suit your specific needs. It is also important that if you are pregnant, under the care of a physician, or suffering from a medical condition, you not take any herbal remedy without first checking with your treating physician or other medical professional. Also see the appendices for information sources and suggested readings.

- Some herbs interact with medications as well as with other herbs. If you are taking conventional drugs, check with a physician, herbalist, or pharmacist who is familiar with both the pharmacology of herbs and of prescription agents before you take an herbal remedy. Also never alter or discontinue any prescription drugs that you are taking without consulting your physician. Herbal manufacturers and their staff researchers may also be able to answer your questions over the telephone.
- Some people believe fresh, freeze-dried herbs contain more of the plant's active ingredients than those that are processed traditionally. This claim has yet to be proved or disproved.
- Some people feel nauseous if they take herbs on an empty stomach. To avoid this, take the remedy after a meal or snack.
- If you experience nausea, diarrhea, or any other unexpected symptom after taking an herb, discontinue taking it and call an expert. You can usually switch to another remedy.

## Types of Herb Formulas

If you prepare your own remedies, always use an enamel, porcelain, or glass container; metal can alter the properties of herbs. Also, never boil herbs.

An *infusion* is made from the soft parts of a plant (leaves, flowers) and is prepared like an herbal *tea,* but is more potent because the herbs are steeped longer than you would for tea. To prepare an infusion: Place ½ to 1 ounce (generally, 1 ounce = 8 teaspoons = 30 grams) of dried or fresh herbs that have been thoroughly bruised in a container. Pour 1 pint of boiling water over the herbs, cover the container tightly, and steep the herbs for 10 to 20 minutes. Strain the liquid and drink the infusion hot, warm, or cool, depending on the herb and the effect you want. The standard dose is 1/2 to 1 cup 3 to 4 times a day, based on the degree of pain. Refrigerate and make a fresh batch daily because herbal infusions decompose rapidly.

A *decoction* is made from roots, stems, and bark. Boil 1 ounce herb to 1 pint water in a covered container for 20 to 30 minutes. Cool and strain. Doses vary from 1 teaspoon to 1 cup taken 3 to 6 times a day. Refrigerate and make a fresh batch daily, as decoctions deteriorate rapidly.

*Extracts* have a higher concentration of active ingredients than infusions and thus are stronger and more effective. The simplest way to make an extract is to thoroughly crush the juicy parts of a plant and press out the juices. For medicinal purposes, 1 ounce of fluid extract is equal to 1 ounce of the pure herb. Refrigerate and make a fresh batch daily.

A *tincture* is an extract made with alcohol instead of water. Because alcohol is a preservative, tinctures can be stored. If you prefer not to use alcohol, apple cider vinegar or wine vinegar work just as well. Tinctures are usually made from potent herbs that are not made into infusions.

Tinctures need 6 weeks to reach full potency. To prepare a tincture at home, steep 1 ounce of dried herb in 5 ounces of vodka, gin, brandy, or grain alcohol or vinegar. Place in a tightly sealed glass container (preferably brown, not clear), label it with the date you prepared it, and store it out of direct sunlight. Shake the container 10 to 100 times every day. If the tincture level goes down, add more alcohol or vinegar to maintain the original level. At six weeks, strain out the plant materials if you desire. When stored in a cool, shaded, or dark place with a tight lid, tinctures can be kept for about one year. The usual dose is 25 drops in water three to four times a day, although this varies depending on the situation.

An herbal *liniment* applied to the back can provide some pain relief. Here's one you might want to try: Combine 2 ounces powdered myrrh, 1 ounce powdered goldenseal (optional), ½ ounce cayenne pepper, and 1 quart rubbing alcohol (70 percent). Mix and let stand for 7 days, giving it a thorough shaking every day. Decant off and bottle in corked bottles. Apply to your back as needed. When stored in a cool, dark, or shaded place with a tight lid, liniments will keep for about a year.

A *compress* made with ginger is effective for relieving chronic muscle tension in the back. Grate ½ pound fresh ginger and place it in a thin cloth that is about 1 foot square (a bandanna is a good size). Tie the opposite corners securely. Place the bag in 2 quarts of heated water and let it sit for 30 minutes. Squeeze the bag to release the ginger juice. Dip a towel into the hot water and wring out the excess liquid. The towel should be as hot as you can tolerate without burning yourself. Place the towel on the tense area of your back. Once it cools, redip it and reapply it several times.

Another soothing experience for back pain is a *mustard pack,* which is used to relieve lower back pain, increase circulation, and ease joint and muscle pain. Visit your local health food store or grocery and buy dry mustard powder and some flour. Mix together 1 tablespoon of the mustard powder, 4 to 8 tablespoons of flour, and a little warm water until it forms a paste. Place the mixture inside a cotton or flannel cloth that has been folded into thirds. Keep the cloth warm by placing it over a food steamer. Spread a little vegetable or olive oil over the area to be treated and place the mustard pack on top. Cover it with a dry cloth and leave it there for at least 10 minutes.

## How to Treat Back Pain with Herbs

Herbal medicine is not a licensed profession in the United States, but there are many trained herbalists you can contact for help in choosing herbal remedies. If you cannot find an herbalist in your area, you can consult with a naturopath or homeopath, as many of them are knowledgeable about herbs. Most people who use herbs are self-taught, using some of the excellent books that have been written on the subject and contacting professional herbal organizations for information (see Appendix A).

Herbs are prescribed based on an individual's symptoms. When taken in the recommended dosages, they are safe and do not cause side effects. The wide variety and versatility of herbs make herbal medicine challenging and offer many different therapeutic combinations. If you purchase commercial herbal remedies, follow the package dosage directions.

Below you will find several herbal recipes for back pain. Following the recipes, you will find an alphabetical list of herbs, their common names, and their indicated uses for back pain and related symptoms. This list is by no means exhaustive but does include popular back-pain remedies.

---

### HERBAL RECIPES FOR BACK-PAIN RELIEF

- For a diuretic tea (see ''Why Use a Diuretic for Back Pain?''), use one part each of juniper berries, uva ursi (bearberry), parsley root, and marshmallow root. Simmer 2 ounces of this herbal mixture in 2 pints of water for 15 minutes in a tightly covered pan. Strain and drink ½ cup three to four times a day.

- For a diuretic-antispasmodic combination, mix 6 parts of Prince's pine and 1 part each of valerian, lobelia, gingerroot, and marshmallow root. Simmer 2 ounces of these herbs in 2 pints of water for 30 minutes and drink 1 cup three times a day or more often until relief is achieved.

- If swelling accompanies your back pain, mix 4 parts echinacea and 1 part lady's slipper. Make a tincture and take 5 to 10 drops every 2 hours. For external relief, apply as a poultice, which you can make by mixing equal parts of comfrey root, horsetail, gravel root, marshmallow root, lobelia, and gingerroot. Simmer 1 ounce of this mixture in 1 pint of water for 30 minutes. Dip red flannel or thick cotton cloth into the solution and apply or wear the cloth to bed as warm as possible each night, using a plastic sheet to protect the bed.

## WHY USE A DIURETIC FOR BACK PAIN?

How can a diuretic herbal remedy help your back pain? According to Michael Tierra, N.D., back pain is often symptomatic of organic (physical) problems, most of which originate from kidney and bladder weakness. This is a belief long held by the Chinese (see "Foods to Enjoy and Foods to Avoid" under "Diet/Nutrition"). Toxins that are normally eliminated through the kidneys and bladder urine are deposited in the surrounding tissues, especially the spinal joints of the lower back. When back pain is accompanied by inflammation, often the nerves have been irritated, and the result is shooting pains called sciatica.

## Herbs for Your Back Pain

### *Arnica (Arnica montana; Arnica fulgens)*

An anti-inflammatory and an analgesic, arnica is applied externally as a liniment for bruises and aches. Arnica is popular and a common part of a natural-remedy first aid kit. Precaution: Some people get a rash from arnica.

### *Cayenne (Capsicum frutescens)*

For chronic pain, apply in a liniment (see "Herbal Recipes" box). Capsicum contains capsaicin, which causes the elimination of a compound (substance P) that mediates the delivery of pain signals from the peripheral nerves to the spinal cord. Precaution: Capsicum can cause skin irritation.

### *Chamomile* (*Matricaria chamomilla,* the German or Hungarian herb; and *Anthemis nobilis,* the Roman or English herb); also called Roman camomile, garden camomile, ground apple

Chamomile (sometimes camomile) is actually two herbs that are botanically unrelated, but they have similar healing properties. Both herbs are anti-inflammatories that help relieve the buildup of tension. As an infusion, mix with equal parts of peppermint and catnip. To prepare an infusion, steep 2 to 3 heaping teaspoons of flowers per cup of boiling water for 10 to 20 minutes and drink up to 3 cups a day. In a tincture, use ½ to 1 teaspoon up to 3 times daily; as an extract, 10 to 20 drops in water up to 3 times daily. Precautions: Do not use chamomile if you have previously reacted to ragweed. If you accidentally consume a large amount of chamomile in a highly concentrated form, you may experience nausea and vomiting.

### Cramp Bark *(Viburnum opulus)*

This is a strong muscle relaxant that can reduce tension in the skeleton and is useful when applied as a hot compress.

### Devil's Claw *(Harpagophytum procumbens);* also called Grapple plant

A standard decoction or tincture of devil's claw can relieve pain and reduce inflammation. It also relieves tension headache and headache that accompanies arthritis and spondylosis. As an added bonus, this plant reportedly lowers cholesterol and fat levels.

### Elderberry *(Sambucus canadensis);* also called pipe tree, popgun tree, common elder

The Native Americans cooked and ate elderberries for back pain, rheumatism, and sciatica. Today elderberry wine is used to treat sciatica. Ten grams of port wine added to 30 grams of elderberry juice is one suggested remedy.

### Goutwort *(Aegopodium podagraria);* also called gout herb, bishopwort

Classified as a diuretic and sedative, it is effective in the treatment of joint aches and pains and for sciatica. Take as an infusion: 4 to 6 ounces 4 to 5 times a day for chronic pain. For acute pain, take every 2 hours until you get relief. If you use the extract, mix ½ teaspoonful in a small glass of water and take 3 times a day. For sciatica, make a poultice. Steep the leaves in hot water and spread them between two pieces of cloth. Lay the cloth on the painful area and place a dry towel on top of the poultice. If you want the poultice to remain hot, use a hot-water bottle instead of a dry towel. Wet the poultice with water as needed; do not let it dry out. Leave the poultice on for several hours if possible. A poultice should be replaced every 3 to 4 hours and reapplied until you get relief.

### Juniper *(Juniperus communis)*

Juniper oil can be added to bath water to soothe muscle pain and arthritic pain. It is also good as a massage oil: dilute 10 drops of juniper oil in 5 ml of almond oil and massage into painful joints. A tea made from the berries, mixed with equal parts of rue, is good for pain.

### Rue *(Ruta graveolens)*

This herb has been used for millennia. Boil 1 pint of water, remove from the heat, and steep a tablespoonful of rue in the water for 30 minutes. Drink ½ cup every 2 to 4 hours. Effective against nervousness and spasms. As a poultice, it is good for sciatica and painful joints. **Caution:** *Rue should not be used during pregnancy.*

### Uva ursi *(Arctostaphylos uva-ursi);* also called bearberry

Uva ursi is often used in combination with other herbs (see "Herbal Recipes") and is taken for urinary tract inflammation and all kidney and bladder problems.

### Valerian *(Valerian officinalis)*

This antispasmodic reduces muscle tension and calms the nerves, which makes it good for insomnia. It also relaxes the blood vessel walls and improves circulation. Use as an infusion (add a few drops of peppermint water or honey to disguise the flavor) for stress and insomnia or as a compress for muscle spasm and cramps.

### Willow Bark *(Salix alba)*

Willow bark is both an anti-inflammatory and an analgesic. In modern herbal practice the bark is the only part usually used. For pain make an extract, tincture, or decoction.

## Where to Get Herbs

Herbal remedies may be derived from herbs, leafy plants, weeds, trees, ferns, or lichens. Different parts of the plant may be used, including the root, bulb, stem, bark, flower, stigma, fruit, seed, resin, or rhizome. Dried herbs, either prepacked or in bulk, are available commercially at health or natural food stores, homeopathic pharmacies, or through a naturopath or mail-order house. A list of commercial suppliers of herbs and remedies appears in Appendix B. If you want to grow and prepare your own herbs and remedies, see "Suggestions for Further Reading" or consult with an herbalist in your area who grows his or her own. A few pots on your porch or a small plot in your vegetable garden is probably all you'll need to keep you well supplied.

## How Does Herbal Medicine Work?

Nature "knows" what works. The active components of each herb—the organic compounds such as enzymes, sugars, vitamins, and proteins—interact in a unique way to treat symptoms and restore the vital force. One example of this synergistic relationship is the meadowsweet plant. This herb contains salicylate compounds like those found in common aspirin. These are the same substances that cause stomach irritation and bleeding in some people. Meadowsweet, however, also contains "associated factors," substances that reduce stomach acidity and soothe the stomach lining. Because herbalists prescribe meadowsweet as a whole herb, pain relief is possible without stomach upset for most people who are sensitive to aspirin.

Unlike homeopathy, in which a single agent is prescribed, herbal medicine uses combinations of plants to create a complete herbal remedy that addresses a person's specific needs. The formulas herbalists and commercial herbal manufacturers use have been handed down through millennia and come from many traditions. Despite the tens of thousands of miles that separated some of the ancient cultures from which the formulas sprung, the similarities in the use of the remedies are remarkable, and those similarities continue today. Another thing that also persists are the common perceptions and goals of the various traditions: that disease results from an imbalance or lack of harmony within the body and that natural healing occurs when an individual's physical, emotional, and spiritual states are aligned for health. When you include herbs in your treatment regimen, you welcome in the opportunity for harmony and pain relief.

## HOMEOPATHY

The basis of homeopathy (*homeo*, "like"; *pathos*, "disease") is the belief that "like may be cured by like." Thus the remedies homeopaths prescribe would, if taken in their original form, produce the same primary symptoms the individual is experiencing. Does that mean the remedy will cause more backache and pain than you already have? Not at all. Homeopathic remedies are chosen—by a homeopath or by the patient—to help stimulate the internal healing energies so that the body can heal itself. The worst thing that can happen after you take a remedy is—nothing. If the remedy you take does not result in improvement after several days, try another one.

There are approximately two thousand homeopathic remedies, of which about one hundred to two hundred are used routinely. Many remedies are derived from plants, which leads some people to think homeopathy and herbal medicine are alike. They are not, however, and you will discover why later in this section. First, however, let's look at how homeopathy can help your back pain.

## Can I Treat My Back Pain Myself?

Many individuals successfully treat their own back pain using homeopathic remedies. We recommend, however, that you consult a professional homeopath for guidance, especially if the pain is chronic or is accompanied by swelling, shooting pains in the legs, or other unusual symptoms. Homeopaths can assess your profile and choose the most appropriate remedy for you. They also know when to alter your prescription based on how you react to a given remedy and which specific lifestyle modifications to suggest as part of your therapy. There are approximately three thousand medical doctors and licensed health care practitioners practicing homeopathy in the United States. *Important:* If you are taking any prescription or other drugs, or are under medical treatment for a specific medical condition, it is essential that you consult with your doctor or appropriate health professional before taking any homeopathic remedy.

## How Do Homeopathic Remedies Work?

Homeopathic remedies are prescribed based on their ability to allow the cause of a symptom to resolve itself. Herbal medicines are also chosen this way. Here is where these two approaches differ, however. Homeopaths will then select a remedy which, if consumed in a normal or large quantity, would cause the same symptoms they want to eliminate. In addition the dose they prescribe will contain only a very minute amount—or perhaps not even a trace—of the remedy. In homeopathy, remedies are more potent the more they are diluted. That is, less is more.

How can that be? When homeopathic remedies are made, one drop of the base formula—the chosen plant part—is mixed with 99 drops of water or alcohol. This is shaken well and then one drop of this mixture is added to 99 drops of water or alcohol and shaken again. This process (called *potentization*) is repeated perhaps hundreds of times. Although it seems the formulation should get weaker each time it is diluted, the opposite is true. The more times a remedy goes through potentization, the greater its power to cure.

"Why?" is the natural response to this statement, and scientists are still looking for the answer. One possible explanation is that, according to quantum physics, all physical substances are composed of energy and leave behind an energy field, like footsteps in the sand, as they move or change position. During repeated potentization no molecules of the original substance may be found in the resulting remedy. However, "footsteps" of the molecules are in these remedies and exist at high energy—and hence high potency—levels.

Thus homeopathy is contrary not only to conventional medicine, in which drugs are given to destroy organisms or suppress symptoms rather than deal with the underlying cause. It is also different from herbal medicine, in that homeopathy is a *bioenergy medicine,* like acupuncture and shiatsu, which manipulate the vital (or life) force, the life energy that connects the physical, emotional, and spiritual part of every person. When your vital force is neglected or blocked, you get symptoms, such as backache or stomach pain. The natural tendency of the vital force is health and balance, and homeopathic remedies allow the force to achieve that goal. Conventional medicine does not recognize this life force because it has not yet "proven" its existence scientifically. Unlike other bioenergy therapies, however, homeopathy involves remedies and their effect on a molecular level, thus it is in a class by itself.

## A Visit with a Homeopath

When you go to a homeopath, expect to spend at least one hour for the first visit. You will be asked questions about your job, social life, hobbies, medical history, and family. Some questions may seem a little odd; for example did you talk in your sleep as a child? are your hands and feet hot or cold at night? All of your answers are important. Homeopaths believe it is essential to have a complete picture of an individual's physical, emotional, and spiritual state—what they call the bodymind—in order to make an accurate diagnosis and choose the best remedy for you. Much of what they learn is done by listening to you and observing your behavior and even how you dress. If they suspect an underlying condition, they may ask you to undergo medical tests (see Chapter 2). All the information they gather helps them develop a personality profile of you.

### HOW TO TAKE HOMEOPATHIC REMEDIES

You can get homeopathic remedies from your practitioner or at a drug or health food store. If you want to make your own remedies, consult with a homeopath or see ''Suggestions for Further Reading'' for a list of books that can help you.

The most common forms of homeopathic remedies are drops or tablets (sugar pills) that have been infused with the remedy. These remedies are prepared by homeopathic pharmacies, which follow the guidelines of the *Homeopathic Pharmacopoeia of the United States,* the official manufacturing manual recognized by the Food and Drug Administration.

If you treat yourself for backache, pick a remedy that best matches your primary general symptoms (see suggestions below). You may have to try more than one remedy before you find one that works for you.

- At least ten but preferably thirty minutes before taking a remedy, do not put anything into your mouth, including food, beverages, gum, mouthwash, toothpaste, or tobacco smoke.
- Avoid taking conventional medicine, such as aspirin, ibuprofen, or laxatives while using a homeopathic remedy. If you are using a prescription medication, consult with your physician before you start the homeopathic remedy or vary any medication.
- Homeopathic drops and tablets are dissolved on or under the tongue so that absorption can occur through the mucous membranes of the mouth. You shouldn't wash them down with water.
- Many homeopaths recommend avoiding coffee, both regular and decaffeinated, during a course of homeopathic treatment. Coffee can cancel out the benefits of many remedies.

## Dosing

"The label on my remedy says 'Belladonna 30c 2h.' What does that mean?" In this example, *30c* is the potency, or strength, of the remedy. The higher the number, the greater the potency. Thus a 30c packs more punch than a 6c. The *c* refers to how the remedy was diluted. The letter *c* refers to the centesimal scale: Thus a 1c remedy was diluted 1:100; a 2c, 1:10,000, and so on. The centesimal scale is the most commonly used system in the United States, and the 6c and 30c dosages are the most widely prescribed. The *2h* means that you should take the remedy every two hours during waking hours.

Both dosages and dosage intervals are highly variable and depend on your particular needs, the individual homeopath, and the manufacturer of the remedy. The ultimate goal of any remedy, however, is to stimulate the healing process just enough to gently restore health.

A few notes about dosing of homeopathic remedies:

• They are highly individualistic, so the remedy that's appropriate for your back pain will probably differ from the one for your spouse or friend who has a similar type of pain.

• Most homeopaths follow a single-remedy approach in which you take only one remedy at a time. If that one does not bring relief, then you stop and take another one.

• The dosages provided in the ''Remedies'' section below are suggestions only; if you don't notice any improvement or you have any questions or concerns, consult a homeopath.

• Occasionally a person may feel worse after taking a remedy. This temporary increase in pain, known as proving, is an indication that a particular remedy *is working*. Not everyone has this reaction, however. The increased pain may last only a few minutes, longer if you are treating chronic pain. Proving may occur if the potency you took was too high for you. Consult with a homeopath or try a lower potency.

• If you start to feel better and stop the remedy but then reach a plateau, restart the remedy at a higher potency. If your worsening pain is accompanied by fever, confusion, or other new symptoms, contact your homeopath or physician immediately.

## Homeopathic Remedies for Your Back Pain

Each of the different types of back pain discussed in this section is followed by a suggested homeopathic remedy. See the "Dosage Guidelines" box for recommended dosages and intervals. Additional information about each remedy is provided under "About the Remedies" immediately following this section.

---

### DOSAGE GUIDELINES

To help you determine how much and how often to take homeopathic remedies, use the Rule of Three, which is summarized below. Generally the more severe the symptoms, the more often you should take the remedy. Always stop and assess your pain after you have taken up to three doses. If you have significant improvement, stop taking the remedy. If you have some improvement, continue dosing as suggested below.

*Severe symptoms:* Take the remedy every thirty to sixty minutes for three doses. If improvement is not significant, repeat as necessary for up to one day until the symptoms become mild or moderate.

*Moderate symptoms:* Take the remedy every three hours for three doses and assess. If necessary, repeat every three hours for up to one day until symptoms improve to mild.

*Mild symptoms:* Take the remedy every six hours for three doses and assess. Repeat as necessary up to ten days until symptoms disappear.

---

## Sciatica

Sciatica can be caused by a prolapsed disk, disk degeneration, osteoarthritis, or ankylosing spondylitis. If the remedies below do not offer improvement, see your doctor or homeopath.

- Burning pain that is worse at night, after resting, or when starting to walk: **Gelsemium 6c**
- Tearing pain made better by heat and movement and made worse by inactivity, cold, and damp: **Rhus tox 6c**; some suggest 30c at onset of pain
- In an elderly or invalid person, pain that is worse at night and aggravated by cold; improves with gentle exercise: **Arsenicum 6c**

## Coccydynia

For this pain at the base of the spine, take the appropriate remedy three times a day for seven days.

- Coccyx pain that was brought on by a fall: **Hypericum 6c**
- Coccyx aches and feels bruised; damp weather makes it feel better: **Causticum 6c**
- Drafts and pressure worsen the pain; presence of constipation: **Silicea 6c**

## Fibrositis

The formation of adhesions between individual muscle fibers is called fibrositis. This condition is usually caused by poor postural habits or habitual strain and stress on the muscles due to either physical or emotional factors. If no muscles are torn, this condition typically clears up within three to four days. The remedy should be taken every three hours for up to two days.

- Pain appears suddenly in dry, cold weather and worsens with movement: **Aconite 30c**
- The muscles feel bruised, movement makes the pain worse, and you may feel irritable and restless: **Arnica 30c**
- Pain in the back, neck, and limbs that gets worse with movement and when exposed to dry, cold east winds but is relieved by pressure: **Bryonia 30c**
- Pain and stiffness worse in cold, dry weather or damp weather, after exercise, and around 4:00 A.M.; pressure seems to help; feel irritable: **Nux 6c**

## Lumbago and General Back Pain

Lumbago (midback pain, just below the waist) is usually caused by overstrenuous activity. Muscles may be strained, torn, or go into spasm, or the ligaments may be torn. Pain may be severe and debilitating and happen suddenly or develop overnight. For pain that comes on suddenly, try one of the following remedies every hour for up to ten doses:

- Sharp pain that worsens when exposed to cold, dry weather and drafts: **Aconite 30c**
- Severe pain that occurs because of injury: **Arnica 30c**

The following remedies can be taken four times daily for up to ten days:

- Lower back feels bruised and stiff, especially in cold, damp weather and after resting; movement reduces the pain: **Rhus tox 6c**
- Back is sensitive to slight touch and feels bruised; pain comes on in cold, dry weather and is made worse by movement: **Bryonia 6c**
- The pain causes restlessness and sleeplessness. The thoracic spine is sensitive to touch: **Cimicifuga 6c**

- Pain is severe, continuous, and dull; aggravated by stooping and walking: **Aesculus 6c**
- Pain worsens with movement or a chill: **Nux 6c**
- Back feels bruised and sore, as above, but is worse from continued motion: **Arnica 30c**

## Osteoarthritis

For chronic osteoarthritis a homeopath can devise a constitutional treatment for you. In cases of acute flare-up pain, the following remedies are suggested, to be taken four times daily for up to two weeks:

- Pain is relieved by heat but worsened by cold and damp, more annoying when inactive but improves with movement; stiffness is worse in the morning: **Rhus tox 6c**
- Severe pain that is relieved by cold applications and worsened by heat and movement: **Bryonia 30c**
- Heat and warm surroundings increase the pain; feel weepy: **Pulsatilla 6c**

## Strained and Pulled Muscles

When overuse or unaccustomed activity tears individual muscle fibers, pain and stiffness result. Immediately after the injury, take **Arnica 30c** every hour up to six times, then four times daily for up to three days. If the pain continues after this, take **Rhus tox 6c** four times daily for up to seven days.

## Ankylosing Spondylitis

Constitutional treatment is recommended. For acute cases of ankylosing spondylitis, the suggested remedy is **Aesculus 6c** taken three times daily for up to five days.

## About the Remedies

Homeopaths use modalities to help them determine which remedy to prescribe. A *modality* refers to the response of a symptom, such as back pain, to external circumstances. For example, is your back pain relieved by (''better for'') heat but worse for cold and damp? Is it worse for inactivity but better for movement? A yes to these questions indicates Rhus tox would be a good choice.

Below are the common name, scientific name, and modalities for the homeopathic remedies suggested in the ''Homeopathic Remedies for Your Back Pain'' section. You can use this information to help you choose the most suitable remedy for your back pain, in conjunction with your health professional, or simply to help you better understand the qualities these remedies possess.

- **Aconite** *(Aconitum napellus)* wolfsbane, blue aconite, blue monkshood

  Aconite depresses the sensory nerve endings. Worse for cold, dry weather and drafts, warm rooms, and lying on the affected side. Better for open air, after sweating, rest.

- **Aesculus** *(Aesculus hippocastanum)* horse chestnut (ripe chestnuts)

  Worse for walking, stooping, cold air, and winter; better for summer and open air.

- **Arnica** *(Arnica montana)* leopard's bane

  Bruises and pain due to falls. Back pain that improves as you start to move but grows worse as movement continues. Better for lying down, clear, cold weather; worse for touch, motion, and heat.

- **Arsenicum** *(Arsenicum album)* arsenic trioxide

Better for warmth, hot drinks; worse for the sight or smell of food, consumption of cold food and drinks; discomfort worse on the right side and between midnight and 2:00 A.M.

- **Bryonia** *(Bryonia alba)* white or common bryony

Activity is in its resin. It acts on the fibrous tissues, ligaments, and serous membranes. Worse for motion, exertion, touch, warmth, sitting. Better for lying down, especially on the painful side, pressure on the pain, quiet, rest, cold drinks, cool air, and applications.

- **Causticum** *(Causticum habnemanni)* potassium hydrate

Worse for cold, dry winds, sweet foods, coffee, grief, heat and humidity, and fright; better for cold drinks and drafts.

- **Cimicifuga** *(Cimicifuga racemosa)* black snakeroot, black cohosh (root or resinoid)

Low back pain that causes restlessness and insomnia. Worse for menstruation; better for warmth.

- **Gelsemium** *(Gelsemium sempervirens)* yellow jasmine

Worse for early in the day and at bedtime, sun, heat, damp, fog, tobacco, emotional stress; better for open air, exercise, passing urine, local heat, bending forward.

- **Hypericum** *(Hypericum perforatum)* St. John's wort

Worse for touch, cold, damp, fog, warm, stuffy rooms; better for tilting the head back.

- **Nux** *(Strychnos nux vomica)* poison nut tree

Backache relieved by sitting up or turning over in bed. Worse for cold wind, dryness, noise, spices, eating, anger, touch, winter; better for warmth, sleep, firm pressure, wet applications.

- **Pulsatilla** *(Pulsatilla nigricans)* wind flower, pasque flower

Low back pain not improved by movement. Worse for sun, heat, temperature changes, rich or fatty foods, lying on the painful side; better for crying, raising the hands above the head, gentle exercise, fresh air, cold drinks, cold applications.

- **Rhus toxicodendron** *(Rhus toxicodendron)* poison ivy

Affects the fibrous tissue—joints, tendons, and sheaths. Important remedy for sprains and strains. Worse for sleep and rest, cold wind, thundery weather; better for warmth, changing position frequently, movement, rubbing.

- **Silicea** *(Silicea terra)* quartz, rock crystal, pure flint

The oxide of silicon; a white, odorless, and tasteless powder that is soluble in water. Usually given for chronic complaints that develop slowly. Worse for morning, dampness, drafts, cold, windy weather, lying on the left; better for summer, warmth.

## What's So Good About Homeopathic Remedies?

One of the best advantages of homeopathic remedies is that, unlike drugs, they do not cause side effects. It may, however, take several doses before you notice results. Chronic backache may take a day or two to subside. Once you start to feel better, you can stop taking the remedy.

Homeopathic remedies are also less expensive than most traditional drugs and often work much more dramatically and rapidly. They are easy to administer and have either a sweet or a slight taste. When you follow the directions of your physician or those on the label, they are a safe, effective alternative to conventional medical treatments.

# HYDROTHERAPY

Water is often referred to as a natural healer, and it can heal in a multitude of ways. Water cleanses and replenishes the body both inside and out. It is responsible for the function and growth of all the cells in the body; it helps maintain body temperature, blood volume levels, muscle strength, digestion, and lubrication of the joints. Without it we would die.

In addition to these wonderful properties, water can also be used to ease pain and even increase mobility. (Water movement routines are discussed in ''Movement Therapy.'') Here are several ways it can be used:

- *Anesthetic:* Ice packs dull pain and reduce painful swelling.
- *Relaxant:* Hot or ice packs, hot and cold compresses, warm baths, and whirlpool can relieve muscle tension and ease pain.
- *Restorative tonic:* When applied as a hot or cold spray or shower, in a whirlpool, or in hot or cold compresses, water increases circulation and stimulates the body's natural healing action.
- *Rubefacient:* Alternating hot and cold water in any form increases circulation in the area treated.

You can also use water as a medium in which to do simple movement routines in the bathtub or hot tub—no swimming pool required! Let's start with these simple routines below. You can incorporate them easily into your bath time. If you don't have a tub, there are several shower and hot and cold applications you can try. (Also see "Thermotherapy" for other heat-related techniques.) Some people add the essential oil of comfrey to their bath or compresses, as this herb soothes aches and pains.

## Bathtub and Hot-tub Movements

The first two movements can be done in the bathtub. Fill the tub to just below underarm level or a bit lower to avoid splashing water over the sides. This level allows water's natural buoyancy to relieve the strain and stress of doing leg lifts. You may need to plug up the overflow drainage hole to keep the water level high. The water should be between 80 and 90 degrees F. Herbal oils in the water can add a calming effect (see "Essential Oils" under "Massage").

### Leg Lifts

Lean back against the back wall of the tub opposite the faucet so that your head is comfortably out of the water and your body is immersed. Hold on to the sides of the tub if you need the support. Inhale and lift one leg out of the water, just above the water line. If this is too high, lift your leg to the water line. Hold it up for about five to eight seconds, then slowly let it down. Repeat with the other leg. Do each leg three to five times. This helps strengthen the thighs.

### Abdominal Tightener

Using the same position as for the leg lifts, bend each knee, one at a time, toward your chest. Only go as far as is comfortable. Repeat this motion five times with each leg.

### Body Twists

This movement should be done in a hot tub in which you can sit on a step or the tub bottom and the water is about midchest high.

Sit and extend your legs out comfortably in front of you, keeping your knees slightly bent. Cup your hands or interlock your fingers. Raise and extend your arms until they are parallel with the tub bottom. While you remain firmly seated, slowly swing your arms to the left and then to the right in a smooth motion and as far as is comfortable. If you experience pain, stop.

If you choose other movements to do in a hot tub, keep these precautions in mind:

- Avoid spending more than fifteen to twenty minutes in water that is between 91 and 95 degrees F, and less time in hotter water. The hot water, combined with movement, places stress on the heart.

- If you have high blood pressure or a heart condition, avoid getting into water that is hotter than 99 degrees F.
- If you feel faint or nauseated while you are in a hot tub, get out immediately.
- Always have someone within shouting distance when you are exercising in a tub or hot tub.

## Whirlpool

A whirlpool combines heat (the water should be about 100 degrees F) and pulsating water to increase circulation, relax, and stretch tight, tense muscles and spasms, and thus relieve minor pain. A whirlpool bath gives your back and entire body a gentle massage and allows you to relax completely. Don't overdo it, however. Spend no more than ten minutes in a whirlpool, and get out sooner if you feel dizzy or faint.

## Alternating Hot and Cold Showers

Few things are more invigorating than alternating hot and cold showers. You might think it's a crazy idea, but it really works to relieve chronic backache, stiff muscles, and minor pain, as well as increase circulation. You can do either a full-body shower or focus the spray on the area that hurts. To use this technique, stand under the hot water for up to one minute (don't burn yourself, just use as hot as is comfortable) and then follow it immediately with a cold spray for thirty seconds. Repeat this cycle at least three times. (Caution: If you have a heart condition, please check with your physician before taking alternating showers.)

## Compresses and Packs

A compress is a piece of soft material, such as cotton or wool, that is moistened with either hot or cold water and applied to the body. Sometimes herbs or essential oils are used in a compress to enhance its healing power.

To make a *hot compress,* take three pieces of soft material, such as cotton or flannel. Fold each cloth into thirds. Boil water, adding herbs or oils if desired, and keep the water hot enough so that you can use it when the first compress becomes cool. Hold either end of the first cloth and dip it into the water. Wring out the center of the cloth and apply the compress to the skin, testing it first to make sure it isn't too hot. Once the cloth feels right, cover it with a second, dry cloth to seal in the heat. Once the wet cloth begins to lose its heat, dip in the third cloth and replace the first one. Make at least three applications. After the last application place a cool cloth over the area for several minutes. Hot compresses increase circulation to the hurting area, reduce muscle spasms, and alleviate pain.

To make a *cold compress,* follow the same procedure except use a basin filled with water and ice cubes. A cold compress reduces swelling and relieves muscle pain and discomfort.

An *ice pack* is used primarily to relieve pain and reduce swelling, so it can be one of your first lines of defense after a back injury. Crushed ice is the easiest form to use in an ice pack. Place the ice in a folded towel or an ice bag; or you can use a commercial ice pack that you keep in the freezer. Leave an ice pack on only until your skin begins to throb; any longer can damage the skin. It is best to hold an ice pack on for a minute or two, take it off, then replace it. Repeat this alternating procedure for no longer than twenty to thirty minutes.

# HYPNOSIS

The hardest part of hypnosis, says Rita Rogers, Ph.D., a hypnotherapist and counselor for nearly forty years, is breaking through people's unrealistic beliefs about hypnosis. Hypnosis is about having control, not losing it, and the work of the hypnotherapist, she says, is to help people understand and use their own power.

Hypnosis is an altered state of awareness, not a loss of consciousness or will, in which a person has an increased capacity to respond to suggestions. Beyond its entertainment value, which is only a very small part of hypnosis, this therapeutic technique helps people reduce pain, quit smoking, lose weight, improve their complexion, and many other healthy changes. Ninety-four percent of patients benefit from hypnosis, even if the only advantage they receive is relaxation. In this section we focus on how you can use self-hypnosis to reduce back pain, stress, and muscle tension.

Self-hypnosis is much more useful—and inexpensive— than returning again and again to a hypnotherapist. Once you learn self-hypnosis, you can practice it anytime you need it and feel secure in doing so.

## Getting Pain Relief with Self-hypnosis

Brian M. Alman, Ph.D., clinical psychologist and author of *Self-Hypnosis for Health and Self-Change,* became interested in self-hypnosis because of his own back pain. He notes that self-hypnosis commonly results in pain relief in the first few sessions, even if the pain is chronic. Four things determine your ability to get pain relief using self-hypnosis: (1) your success in developing a self-hypnotic trance; (2) how motivated you are to get pain relief; (3) how well you are able to let go of your fear of releasing your pain; and (4) understanding that you have control over your pain. Let's look at each point briefly:

1. This takes practice. Period. Relaxation is your first goal, as release of muscle tension often alleviates some pain immediately. Then you can deal directly with your pain. We look at a self-hypnosis technique below.

2. You may think it's unusual that someone wouldn't be motivated to get rid of his or her pain, but sometimes people have an unconscious reason to want to keep hurting. Perhaps it prevents them from returning to a job they don't like; maybe they're collecting workman's compensation; or they may like getting sympathy. For self-hypnosis to work, you need to *want* to feel better.

3. "What if I hypnotize my pain away completely and I hurt myself because I can't feel anything?" Self-hypnosis only reduces unnecessary pain, and this selective feature makes self-hypnosis a good pain-relief technique. Pain is a signal that something is wrong. When you take painkillers, you run the risk of covering up all those signals, even the ones that alert you that something serious or new is amiss. Drugs can also make you feel less alert or drowsy (see the discussion of drugs and their side effects in Part III). According to Dr. Alman, "it is very important . . . not to try eliminating all pain, but to be selective. With self-hypnosis you can learn to control unwanted, unnecessary pain, but still experience any new sensation that is alerting you to a new problem or a change in the existing one."

4. Even though the pain originates somewhere in your back or is referred to your back, the mind interprets the pain. Understanding that the mind is an extraordi-

nary tool and that you can control your pain is very empowering. "What finally made self-hypnosis work for me was when I realized that I had the power to control my back pain," said Steven, a thirty-seven-year-old management consultant who suffered with daily back pain for four years before he tried self-hypnosis. He was skeptical at first, but he was strongly motivated to try anything besides the pain-killers he had been taking, which sometimes affected his concentration and no longer gave him much relief. He worked with a hypnotherapist who helped him choose suggestions to control his pain. Steven has tapes of some of his sessions and he uses these or his own self-hypnosis routine every day and has significantly reduced his pain to the point where he can play tennis again.

## How Does Hypnosis Work?

Hypnosis helps you separate the sensation of pain from the discomfort and awful feeling that accompany it. Drs. Ronald Melzack and Patrick D. Wall, who are well known for their research of pain, explain how self-hypnosis works: "It changes the way you feel pain. You can turn off the region that feels the awfulness, the unpleasantness, yet you still sense and describe the pain—where it is and what it is, without feeling the discomfort from it."

You can achieve this separation using one or more self-hypnosis techniques. These approaches include self-hypnosis through progressive relaxation, eye fixation, indirect language, direct language, dreams, music, time regression, and guided imagery, among others. One very effective way to learn self-hypnosis is to work with a hypnotherapist who can show you the ropes. The therapist can tape your sessions so that you can use them at home.

You can also purchase professionally made self-help tapes or make tapes yourself using scripts that are available either in books or those you make up yourself. Or you can customize prepared scripts to your own particular needs (see *Self-Hypnosis: The Complete Manual* by Brian Alman and Peter Lambrou; also see Appendix B for sources of self-hypnosis tapes).

Preparing for a Self-hypnotic Session

The following guidelines can help you prepare for your self-hypnotic sessions. These are "generic" steps and are followed by instructions for a specific type of hypnotic technique—distraction—which is commonly used for pain relief.

- Begin by choosing a comfortable, quiet location where you will not be disturbed for at least twenty-five to thirty minutes. During your first few sessions it will probably take you up to fifteen minutes to fully enter a hypnotic state and focus on your goals. Once you are adept at relaxing and entering a trance, your entire session can last as little as eight to ten minutes.
- "Should I sit or lie down?" It's your choice; do what is most comfortable for you. If you are in pain, get into a position that minimizes it.
- "Should I close my eyes?" Many people close them once they are in the hypnotic state because it helps them visualize and focus more clearly. If keeping them open works for you, do it.
- Proper breathing is key. Refer to "Breathing Therapy" for guidelines on deep breathing. This is an excellent way to begin your session because it relaxes your body and helps clear the mind so that you can more easily enter the hypnotic state.

- Once you are comfortable and have taken a few deep breaths, fix your eyes on an object or spot that is in front of you and above your line of vision. It can be anything simple: a flower, a stain on the wall, or a glass on the counter. Keep your attention focused on the spot you have chosen and continue to breathe slowly and deeply. Prompt yourself to relax using suggestions such as *"With every breath I let out I feel tension and worry leave my body. The more I relax, the better I feel."* Use whatever words or phrases you want; the goal is to relax and let your mind be free of extraneous thoughts. Also give yourself suggestions to close your eyes. *"My eyes feel heavy; I welcome the comforting feeling of having my eyes closed."* Even after your eyes are closed, keep reinforcing the relaxation you feel.

## Distraction for Pain Relief

When you use *distraction,* you focus your attention on places on your body that are not in pain. After you have completed the "Preparing for a Self-hypnotic Session" guidelines, select a part of your body that is pain-free and comfortable, say, your foot. Concentrate on it; picture it in your mind. Reinforce how good it feels. Give yourself suggestions for pain relief and make them positive. For example *"As I concentrate on my foot and notice how relaxed it feels, how comfortable it feels, I may begin to notice a lightness and warmth in my toes. The feeling is pleasant, and I will remain focused on that feeling for as long as it lasts, whether it's a few seconds or a few minutes."* During this time of intense concentration you distract yourself from the pain in your back to a pleasant feeling in your foot. Move on to other body parts and repeat the process, or remain focused on the foot; it is up to you.

The first time Claudia tried distraction, she got "only ten seconds of relief." The next day she tried again and found that by going in and out of a trance several times in a row, she had better control. Her persistence has paid off. After several weeks of daily repeat sessions she has extended the distraction time. She added visualization, which has helped her not only to distract from the pain but also to enter a trance faster and stay there longer. Now when Claudia focuses on her feet, for example, she visualizes splashing them in a cool pool of water or having someone massage them, two images that work well for her.

# MASSAGE

*The physician must be experienced in many things, but most assuredly in rubbing . . . for rubbing can bind a joint that is too loose and loosen a joint that is too rigid.*

—*Hippocrates*

Massage is one of the most relaxing therapies a person can experience. A good back massage does more than relax you; it can stimulate circulation, which helps flush waste materials out of the hurting muscles. Massage also reportedly helps strengthen the body's resistance to disease by improving overall physical condition. If you are in the throes of acute pain and are contemplating massage, we recommend that you have a professional do it. If you have discomfort or are not in pain, massage is an excellent activity for you and a friend or partner to learn together. Naturally the person who has the aching back gets treated first!

There are many types and variations of massage—deep muscle, Esalen, Hawaiian, Oriental, sport, Swedish, and more—too many to address individually in this book. Our purpose here is to introduce you to the basics of massage, explain how you can do self-massage, and provide easy instructions for a partner to do massage for you. The "Suggestions for Further Reading" section offers the names of books on various types of massage you can explore.

## Self-massage

Massaging your own back can be done with one or two inexpensive devices, including a tennis ball or softer rubber ball, or a tubelike roller. The roller consists of a six-inch-diameter piece of Ethafoam cylinder that is about three feet long. You may be able to get a piece from a packaging business, or you can order a roller from a physical therapy and medical supply store (see Appendix B). You can also make your own back roller (see box).

---

To make your own back roller for self-massage, you need:

- A one-inch-thick round wooden dowel or hard rubber tube about one foot long
- One large, thick towel (bath size)
- Two twenty-four-inch-long pieces of heavy string or ribbon

Lay the towel flat on the floor and fold the two outer edges in toward the center of the towel. Lay the dowel or tube at one end of the folded towel and roll the dowel up into the towel until you reach the end of the towel. Tie a string around the towel near each end. It's ready to use as a self-massage tool.

---

The massage techniques explained below should not be attempted if you are in a great deal of pain. Stop any massage that causes you discomfort beyond what you have been experiencing daily.

- *For the lower back:* Lie on the floor with your legs bent and your feet flat on the ground. Place a tennis ball under the area you want to massage. Some people find a tennis ball is a bit too hard, so they use a softer, rubber ball that is about the same size. Place as much of your body weight on the ball as is comfortable and rock back and forth.
- *For the upper back:* Starting in the same position as above, place the roller directly under your upper shoulders. Extend your neck back and lift your buttocks off the floor as you roll slowly back and forth. Place your hands on your lower abdomen or on the floor next to you if you need to balance yourself. Do not roll lower than the bottom of your rib cage. Keep the motion small.
- *For the middle back:* Start in the same position as above. Place the roller under your back at mid rib cage. Keep your abdominal muscles firm and your back flat; do not arch. Roll from your mid rib cage to your lower back, slowly and gently. You can lean to either side to work any particular area more than another.

## Partner Massage

Here are a couple of massage routines for your partner to do for you. The instructions are written for and directed to your partner. Remember, with massage, the muscles should be worked deeply but not to the point of pain. Let your partner know if you are not comfortable or feel pain.

## Variation 1

- Avoid placing pressure directly on the spine. This is important for any massage you do on people with back pain.

- Kneel at your partner's head and place your palms flat on either side of the spine just below the neck. Using light pressure, stroke straight down the back to the hips, keeping your fingers together and your fingertips on the back. (Beware of long fingernails. Keep your nails short, or keep your fingertips raised slightly to avoid hurting your partner.) Stroke gently as you bring your hands back to the neck. Repeat the stroke to the hips, applying a bit more pressure this time if your partner is comfortable with it. Complete five of these cycles.

- Return to the base of your partner's neck and place your thumbs on either side. Spread open your fingers and stroke outward and back along the top of the shoulders. Repeat five times.

- Move to your partner's legs and straddle them. Place your thumbs on either side of the spine at its base (the sacrum). Spread your fingers and rotate your thumbs in small circles, slowly massaging the entire lower back on both sides of the spine.

- Now kneel at your partner's side. Place one hand on the far side of the spine at the base of the neck and rest the other on the upper back for support. Using the hand farthest from you, rotate your palm in small circles and push the muscle away from the spine. Work your way slowly down to the buttocks. Return to the base of the neck and repeat the massage two more times. To do the other side, kneel on the other side of your partner and repeat the massage sequence.

- If any of these sequences was particularly soothing or

helpful, repeat it. Likewise, skip any that was uncomfortable.

## Variation 2

- Kneel at your partner's side. Place one hand on top of the other and press with your palms as you make broad circles around the shoulder blade. Do not press directly on the bone or the spine. Repeat five times and then switch shoulders.
- Place your hands on either side of your partner's waist (both of your hands with fingers pointed away from you). Press with your palms as you bring your hands toward each other. As your hands cross over the spine, avoid pressure on the spine. Your hands will end up in the opposite position from where you placed them originally. Repeat this massage motion again just above the first spot. Continue up the back to the shoulders, then repeat the entire routine twice.

## Miscellaneous Variations

These massage methods are from the Chinese and are good for the lower back.

- *Palm Rub:* Lay your palm flat on your partner's back. Rub slowly in a clockwise direction, keeping even pressure.
- *Palm-Heel Rub:* A variation of the palm rub. Apply pressure using the muscular pads on either side of the base of your palm. Keep your fingers and thumb raised off the skin. As you apply forward pressure, rapidly swing your palm left and right from the wrist. Try to reach a rate of 100 to 200 times a minute.
- *Palm-Edge Chafe:* Your partner can sit or lie down for this massage. Using the outer edge of your palm, go up and down both sides of the back with a rapid sawing

motion, more than 100 times a minute if possible. Do this massage with one hand.

## Oils and Ice

An herbal massage oil can make massage even more pleasant. See the accompanying box for some suggestions. If you have pain but no swelling, you may benefit from a brief ice massage. Keep water frozen in paper or Styrofoam cups in the freezer. Your partner can massage the painful area with a circular motion, using the open end of the cup, until the area is numb. Do not use ice for longer than ten minutes.

---

**ESSENTIAL OILS FOR MASSAGE**

*Essential Oils*

- Black pepper (stimulates blood flow; use in small amounts)
- Chamomile (German or Roman; soothes muscular sprains and aches and swollen joints; mixes well with lavender)
- Eucalyptus (cool to the skin but warm to the muscles; mixes well with lavender and juniper)
- Juniper (effective for rheumatism and sports aches and pains; mixes well with rosemary and citrus oils)
- Lavender (an analgesic and antispasmodic; mixes well with citrus oils and frankincense)
- Orange (eases stress; mixes well with juniper and frankincense)
- Rosemary (stimulates circulation and helps ease pain; mixes well with juniper).

  Examples: Combine 5 drops of lavender, 2 each of frankincense and rosemary; use a carrier oil of 20 ml of sweet almond. Combine up to four essential oils from those suggested—choose those that smell best to you—and blend with a carrier oil that suits your skin type.

*Carrier Oils*

- All-purpose oils: apricot kernel oil (light and high penetration); grapeseed and soy (both good for oily skin); sunflower (contains vitamin E); and sweet almond (soothing; good for babies).
- Special carrier oils, which are good for dry, dehydrated skin, can be added to all-purpose oils: carrot (use only enough to make up 10 percent of total mixture; i.e., one drop in ten to be carrot); sesame (do not use the brown oil from the toasted seed); avocado (excellent skin softener); jojoba (nonoily softening action); and wheat germ (strong smell). Benefits of essential oils: anti-inflammatory and warming oils help relax aching muscles.
- Blending and using oils: For a normal dilution of 2.5 percent, the formula is 1 ml of carrier oil divided by 2 equals total drops of essential oil needed. For example: 20 ml carrier oil/2 = 10 drops essential oil. Essential oils evaporate easily and are very sensitive to light and temperature. Always mix and store your oils in a dark bottle and keep them in a cool, dark place. Label and date the bottles, and keep them away from children.
- Ginger: A popular massage medium used by the Chinese is ginger. Use a mortar and pestle or a food processor to reduce fresh gingerroot to a mudlike consistency. Dip your fingers into the juice and apply it to the skin. Ginger juice radiates warmth and makes for a very soothing massage.

# MEDITATION

*Meditation is not a means to an end. It is both the means and the end.*

—*J. Krishnamurti*

Meditation is practiced by millions of people around the world, from all walks of life and for a variety of reasons. Bernie Siegel, M.D., who has done much research on meditation, defines it as "an active process of focusing the mind into a state of relaxed awareness." There are many ways to achieve this, and he goes on to say that regardless of the path one takes, "the result of all meditation methods is ultimately the same: to induce a restful trance which strengthens the mind by freeing it from its accustomed turmoil."

Meditation also has many medical benefits, as much research has shown (see box). Studies by Dr. Deepak Chopra, Dr. Herbert Benson, Dr. Jon Kabat-Zinn, Dr. Bernie Siegel, and others have shown, for example, that meditation lowers or normalizes the levels of stress hormones in the blood and evokes the relaxation response, a state of being in which the mind is quiet and cleared of activity and the body responds with a lower heart and breathing rate, reduced blood pressure, and less oxygen consumption. Once tension is released, many of the body's aches and pains often either disappear or lessen.

---

**BENEFITS OF MEDITATION**

- Reduces lactate levels in the blood (lactate is related to high levels of anxiety)
- Induces the relaxation response

- Increases alpha brain-wave activity—the brain waves present during deep relaxation and creativity
- Decreases the levels of stress hormones in the bloodstream
- Reduces or normalizes blood pressure (recommended as the first line of therapy for mild hypertension)
- Reduces pulse rate
- Improves immune system resistance
- Evidence that over time, it can increase memory, intelligence, creativity, and concentration

There are two basic approaches to meditation: concentrative and mindfulness. In concentrative meditation you focus your attention on your breath, an image, a sound (such as a mantra)—anything repetitive—in order to still your mind and allow greater awareness. This form of meditation was first studied scientifically by Drs. Herbert Benson and R. Keith Wallace, who proved that concentrative meditation decreases heart rate, breathing rate, and oxygen consumption. These changes often occur after only a few weeks of practice.

Mindfulness, according to Joan Borysenko, Ph.D., "involves opening the attention to become aware of the continuously passing parade of sensations and feelings . . . without becoming involved in thinking about them." Don't think? Even skilled meditators think; they just acknowledge it. "Oops, thinking again," they say to themselves, and let it go. Dr. Benson encourages his patients to take such an "Oh, well" attitude toward thinking during meditation. In fact every time you drift into thought and then return to concentration, you strengthen your "mental muscles of awareness and choice," says Borysenko, who sees this action as mental exercise. Indeed meditation is like physical exercise in that when you stop meditation, the physical benefits usually disappear within a few weeks.

## Meditation for Your Back Pain

Here are two meditations for you to try. The first is an example of concentrative meditation and can help strengthen the spine. In as little as eight to ten minutes per day, you can bring yourself to a place of peace and reduced pain. The second is an example of mindfulness of pain and tension. Some people find it helpful to tape meditations they find in books so that they can just pop a cassette into their tape recorder and play the meditation of their choice. You can also purchase prerecorded meditations (see Appendix B).

### *Concentrative Meditation*

1. Choose a comfortable chair and sit with your spine held straight and your eyes closed.
2. Relax your shoulders, lift your chest, and let your chin fall lightly toward your throat. This lengthens the back of your neck.
3. Place your hands on your knees, palms up. If you choose, connect the tips of your thumb and index finger of each hand.
4. Inhale deeply through your nose and slowly exhale. After each exhale squeeze your buttocks and hold this position for a few seconds. Continue deep breathing and squeezing for about two minutes. Concentrate only on your breath and on the squeeze.
5. After two minutes switch your focus to your spine. Meditate on your spine as you breathe deeply into your abdomen. Visualize your spine as you hold it straight and relaxed. Continue to meditate on your spine and breathe deeply for about two minutes.

### *Mindfulness Meditation*

1. Lie down in a comfortable position and slowly stretch so that you feel fully present in your body. Briefly "check in" with your body parts as you stretch, starting with your toes and moving quickly upward until you reach the top of your head.
2. Allow your eyes to close; take a deep breath and slowly exhale.
3. With your next breath shift your breathing to your belly or a spot just below your navel. Let your breath come and go from that place, gently and slowly. Allow yourself to be fully aware of your breathing as it flows in waves.
4. Now allow yourself to shift your focus and to become aware of your body. Choose the painful or tight area in your back and imagine that you can send your breath to that spot. As you breathe in, be aware of any sensations in the area. You can do this without judging whether these sensations are good or bad . . . they simply exist.
5. As you breathe out, notice if the feelings change or shift. Let your breath wash over the pain gently. Acknowledge the sensations and be present with them and let them just be. Continue breathing in and out and allowing the waves of breath to wash over all the sensations you are experiencing.
6. When you feel ready to return, open your eyes and take a slow, deep breath and release it slowly.

With mindfulness meditation you may notice that your pain intensifies at first because you send your awareness to it. As you continue to meditate, however, the pain usually shifts, decreases, or even disappears. It may take several sessions for you to notice a significant difference in your level of pain.

## How Does Meditation Work to Relieve Pain?

Pain has two components: the physical sensations and your thoughts about them. Meditation allows you to change your perception of pain and thus your thoughts about it. At the same time meditation is a discipline and a way of life. The purpose of meditation is to learn how to be without purpose; meditation is about being and not about doing. One result of being is that it brings about an internal quiet that helps regulate the body's metabolic rate and allows the entire central nervous system, which includes the spinal cord, an opportunity to rest. These results can be long-lasting and far-reaching, and they take time to become apparent. That's not to say you won't feel better after just one session—chances are you will.

If you have chronic pain, meditation can be a very welcome addition to your day. According to Dr. Jon Kabat-Zinn, 72 percent of patients with chronic pain achieved at least 33 percent reduction after an eight-week period of mindfulness meditation; 61 percent achieved at least 50 percent reduction.

Meditation works best when you establish a routine; say, twenty minutes of meditation in the morning when you first get up or twenty minutes when you get home at night. Like learning to play the piano, daily meditation practice is important . . . and rewarding. See "Suggestions for Further Reading" for books that give examples of meditation techniques.

## MOVEMENT THERAPY

For years many physicians prescribed long-term bed rest for back pain. But recent research and countless studies have shown that people with back injury should be active almost immediately after the pain-causing event—two days of rest and then *move*! Too much rest weakens the muscles and delays recovery and also tends to make individuals anxious about their pain. And forget the ''E[xercise]''-word— sounds too much like drudgery. You are going to *move* for your health.

Long before the movement approach was accepted by the medical community, Dr. Stephen H. Hochschuler, an orthopedic surgeon specializing in spine surgery and cofounder of the Texas Back Institute, advocated and encouraged patients to be active right after a back injury. Why? Because he knew that movement ''is the best way to centralize the pain from a broad area to a localized area, reduce pain, accelerate the healing process, and lastly prevent the injury from happening again.'' Sound like a good deal? There's more.

Daily movement routines stimulate production of the body's natural painkillers, *endorphins* and *enkephalins,* and also builds strength, flexibility, and endurance, all of which are essential to maintain a healthy back. Add some aerobic activity (see page 175)—once your back is up to it—three to five times a week, and you have a prescription for a healthy back.

There is much discussion about the ''best'' movement program for individuals with low back pain. While trying not to get too technical (refer to Figures I-1 and I-2 when we do), we briefly mention two major types of movements—flexion and extensor—and the indications for each (see box, page 167). Flexion movements open up the intervertebral foramina and facet joints, stretch the hip and back flexor muscles, and strengthen abdominal and gluteal (buttock) muscles. Extension movements are done to improve mobility and endurance and to strengthen the back extensors. Examples of each type of movement are given below. We recommend you work with your physician or other health professional to create a movement program that is designed with your specific condition and needs in mind. When you do start your program, remember the following general guidelines:

- Take it *slow*. Your movements should be graceful and nonstressful. *Ease* into a position; do not strain or use any jolting or jarring motions.
- This is not a contest, so if you can only do one or two repetitions of a given movement, fine. The next time try to increase it by one or two. Eventually you will be strong and flexible enough to do more, although ten to twelve repetitions of any movement is usually considered adequate.
- Be aware of your posture and relax. Tense muscles work against you, not for you.
- Keep your mind free and calm. You might want to practice meditation (see page 162) before starting your movement program.
- Pick movements that you enjoy. Whichever ones you choose, either from those explained here, others you read about, or movements suggested by your health professional, they are most effective if practiced every day. Make them a part of your daily routine, just like brushing your teeth, and you will be more likely to do them. If playing music helps make them more enjoyable, do it!
- When you do a movement that stretches your spine in any one direction, the next movement you do should stretch your spine in the opposite direction. This helps keep your body in balance.
- Do your movement program when it works best for you: some people break up their routine and do five or ten minutes of movements twice a day; others do them before each meal; or perhaps you want to do them all at one time.

- You may feel some minor discomfort when doing the movements and activities the first few times, especially if you are not used to much activity. This is normal, and most people work through it. If any movement causes your back to hurt even more, however, stop doing it. Generally people recognize the full benefit of improved strength and flexibility after the first few movement sessions, which typically are the more painful ones.

---

### WHEN TO DO FLEXION MOVEMENTS

Do flexion movement if your pain is *relieved* when you

- Sit
- Repeatedly bend forward
- Increase swayback (lordosis) of the lower back

*Or* if your pain *worsens* when you

- Walk
- Stand
- Bend forward for an extended time
- Repeatedly bend backward
- Bend backward for an extended time

### WHEN TO DO EXTENSION MOVEMENTS

Do extension movements if your pain is *relieved* when you

- Lie down
- Walk
- Repeatedly bend backward
- Decrease swayback of the lower back

---

*Or* if your pain *worsens* when you

- Sit
- Drive
- Rise from a seated position
- Stoop
- Bend forward
- Repeatedly bend forward

(Adapted from David Borenstein et al., *Low Back Pain: Medical Diagnosis and Comprehensive Management*)

Here are three strengthening movements for the lower back. If possible, do them twice a day.

- **Bent-Knee Situps (Flexor):** Lie on your back with knees bent. With arms extended toward your knees, slowly move toward a situp position. You do not have to actually sit up; simply lift your head and shoulders off the floor. When your stomach muscles are strengthened, you can cross your arms in front of your chest and do the situp. This movement strengthens the abdominal muscles (see Figure II-9).
- **Pelvic Tilt (Flexor):** Lie on the floor with your arms relaxed at your sides. Bend your knees and put your feet flat on the floor. Tighten your buttocks, pull in your abdominal muscles, and tilt your pelvis up so that the small of your back is flattened into the floor. Your abdominal muscles and buttocks should be doing the work—not your arms, feet, or hips. Hold this position for a count of 5 to 10, but don't hold your breath. Relax your muscles as you inhale and return to your starting position. Repeat ten times. This movement strengthens the upper abdominals (see Figure II-10).

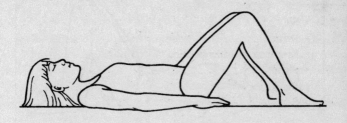

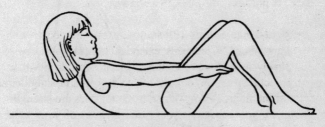

**II-9  Bent-knee situps**

- **Wall Press (Flexor):** Stand with your back, shoulders, and buttocks flat against a wall. While keeping this position, move your feet away from the wall about ten to twelve inches. Slide down the wall slowly until your knees and thighs are at about a 45-degree angle. If your knees hurt at this point, stop the movement. If not, slide down farther until your knees are at a 90-degree angle. Hold this position for no more than fifteen seconds, then slowly rise to a full stand-

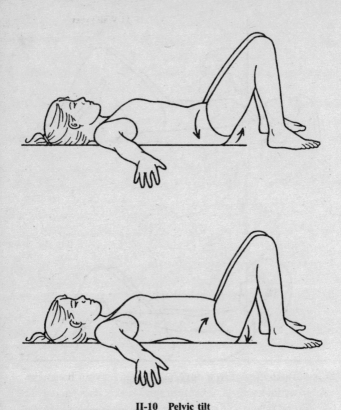

**II-10   Pelvic tilt**

ing position. Repeat two to three times; eventually try to do up to ten. This movement strengthens the quadriceps (muscles in the front of the thighs) (see Figure II-11).

In addition to strong muscles, you also need flexible ones to ward off back pain. Here are two stretching movements to get you started:

**II–11 Wall press**

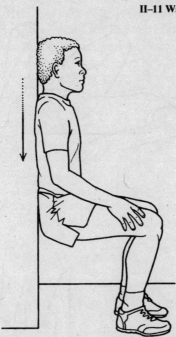

- **Hamstring Stretch (Extensor):** Lie on your back with your knees bent, your feet flat on the floor, and your arms relaxed at your sides. Raise your right knee toward your chest. Straighten and extend the right leg so that it is at about a 45-degree angle with your body. Then *slowly* raise your right leg until it is at a 90-degree angle with your body. Keep your knee straight. Hold this position for a second or two and then return the right leg to the starting position. Repeat the movement with the left leg. When you have completed one full cycle (both legs), repeat the cycle again, up to ten times, when you are able (see Figure II-12).
- **Squeeze and Spread (Extensor):** Here is a two-for-

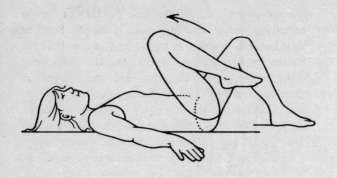

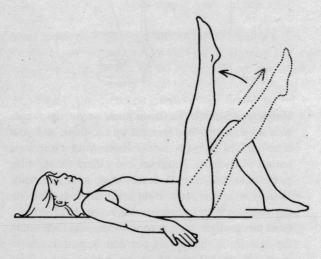

**II-12 Hamstring stretch**

one movement. Start in the same position as for the hamstring stretch. The first move is simple: Squeeze your buttocks together as tightly as you can, hold for five to ten seconds, and then relax. The lower back depends on strong buttocks, and this movement strengthens them. (You can do this part of the Squeeze and Spread movement anywhere—you don't need to lie down. Do it in the office, at a stop light, right now!) The Spread part of the movement is done from the same starting position. Then, without applying or expending any effort, allow your knees to spread apart. When you feel some resistance, hold your legs in that position for a few seconds. Then return to the starting position. Repeat as you are comfortable. The Spread movement stretches the muscles of your groin, buttocks, and hips (see Figure II-13).

Lest you think we forgot those of you with upper back and neck pain, here are two movements for you. Both of them stretch the muscles in the shoulders and upper back.

- **Prone Shoulder Stretch:** Begin in the Hamstring Stretch position. Then slowly raise your right arm straight up to a 90-degree angle and continue to move it until it is extended behind you. Keep your palm up. Remain in that position for about ten seconds and then slowly bring your arm back to your side by reversing the movement. Repeat this sequence with the left arm. Alternate arms several times (see Figure II-14).
- **Shoulder Shrug:** You can do this movement while sitting at a traffic light, lying in bed, watching television—just about anywhere! To begin, raise your shoulders slowly and steadily into a shrug. Hold this position for about ten seconds. Without moving your head, gently press your shoulders down as far as you

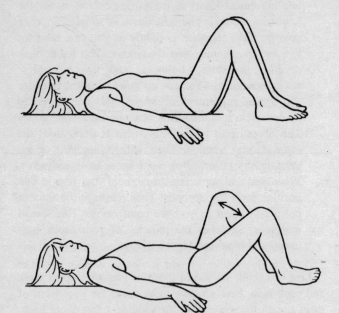

**II-13   Squeeze and spread**

can comfortably. Hold this position for about ten seconds. Feel the muscles stretch in your neck. Now relax
your neck and shoulders. Repeat the Shoulder Shrug
several times (see Figure II-15).

## Aerobic Activities and Sports

Aerobic activity is good for more than your heart and
circulatory system; it also increases the blood flow to the
disks and aids in the healing process. We aren't suggesting
you go jogging the day after a back-pain episode—please

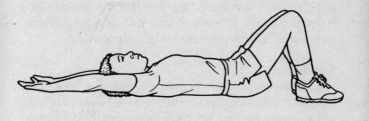

**II-14   Prone shoulder stretch**

don't! Depending on your level of recovery as you do your daily movement routines and increase your muscle strength and flexibility, you can begin or restart aerobic activities

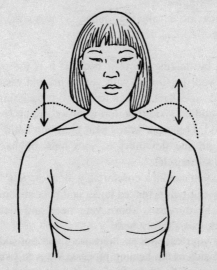

**II-15   Shoulder shrug**

soon after your back-pain episode subsides. Both walking and swimming are generally considered the best aerobic activities for most people with back pain. Bicycling (if you maintain an upright position) is also recommended.

## Swimming

For those with access to a pool, the water provides a safe, nonstressful environment in which to do an aerobic workout and strengthening and flexibility movements. Water eliminates much of the effects of gravity, offers gentle resistance, prevents sudden movements, and reduces stress. Swimming also requires shortening of the back muscles, which strengthens them. A straight leg kick also works the back muscles, but it is recommended that you use a bent leg kick (as explained below) while you are healing. During your first few times in the water you may want to use a flotation device, especially if your back is very sore or you are not a swimmer.

If you decide to take the plunge (so to speak), here are some tips:

- Start by floating on your back. If it is too painful to kick your legs, scull with your arms and wear a flotation device. Kicking can irritate your back muscles, so only add a kicking motion when you're up to it. Once you do, keep your knees bent until you build up more strength and flexibility in your hips, thighs, and abdominal muscles.
- Once you can kick comfortably, float on your back and keep your pelvis tucked under and your abdomen tight. Stretch your arms above your head and kick gently, with knees slightly bent.
- Once your strength has improved, you can add the elementary backstroke and the backstroke. Save the crawl for later, and add the breaststroke, which increases the

arch of the back even more than the crawl does, only if it does not bother your back.

- Try to make fifteen minutes of continuous swimming, three times a week, your goal.

## Swimming with Special Back Problems

If you have a specific back condition, such as scoliosis, spondylolisthesis, or spondylolysis, work with a physical therapist to establish a safe swimming program for you. Here are some guidelines to consider:

- If you have spondylolysis, avoid any movements that cause hyperextension of the spine, including the butterfly, breaststroke, and backstroke. The sidestroke is safe, as are movements that strengthen the abdominal muscles.
- The recommendations for spondylolisthesis are the same as those for spondylolysis, plus you can add water jogging.
- If you have scoliosis, movements that strengthen the entire trunk are recommended. A physical therapist or other knowledgeable health care professional can create a water program that is specific to your needs.

## Water Movements

Because everyone reading this book has a different level of both pain and ability, the water movements suggested in the accompanying box are at the beginner level. All are designed to strengthen and stabilize the trunk and are considered safe and appropriate for most back problems, including herniated disk. For more advanced movements, see "Suggestions for Further Reading" or ask your health care professional.

## BEGINNER-LEVEL WATER MOVEMENTS

NOTE: Do these movements in water that is chest or above-the-waist high.

- *Water Walking:* Begin at one end of the pool and walk across the pool as you would on land: arms swinging, hips pointed straight ahead, and head held high. When you reach the other side, walk backward to the starting point, keeping your legs stiff and knees straight. If walking backward in this way bothers your lower back, take smaller steps and bend your legs. Stop walking backward if you have increased sharp lower back or leg pain.

  Walking backward requires you to use the muscles in the back of your legs—the hamstrings and hip extensors—and you may need to work up to this activity. Do as much as you can and add to this part of your program each time you are in the water. Your goal is eight to ten minutes of water walking.

- *Sideways Walk:* In chest-high water stand along the side of the pool wall and walk sideways by extending one leg to the side and then bringing your other leg to meet it. Keep repeating this movement. When you reach the other side of the pool, simply reverse your steps. Cross the pool several times in this way. This movement improves overall flexibility and works each side of the hips, legs, and trunk independently.

- *Water Kicks:* Stand perpendicular to the side of the pool and hold on to the side with your arm extended. Slowly raise up the leg farthest from the wall only as far as is comfortable. Keep your knee locked, your back straight, and your opposite leg straight with the heel down. Do not lean forward or backward when you kick. After you kick forward, bring your leg backward in one smooth motion and extend it behind you twelve to eighteen inches, or whatever is comfortable for you. Repeat the forward kick and backward motion several times, with your eventual goal being twenty or thirty times. When you complete one side, turn around and do the other leg.

- *Trunk Twisting:* (You need a kickboard or a large floating barbell for this movement.) Stand more than arm's-length away from the side of the pool and with your feet shoulder-width apart and pointing straight ahead. While holding a barbell or kickboard at each end, slowly and evenly twist from side to side as far as is comfortable. Keep your elbows locked and your heels flat. This flexibility movement is good for chronic pain.

- *Barbell Push and Pull:* (You need two hand barbells or two large empty plastic milk jugs for this movement.) Stand with your feet shoulder-width apart and pointing straight ahead. Hold a dumbbell or jug in each hand with the palms up. Push the weights away from you in a straight line and then pull them back toward you. Repeat this movement twenty to thirty times without stopping. This movement improves upper-back posture and builds up endurance and upper-body strength. If you cannot do both arms together, alternate them and increase the number of repetitions if possible. Throughout the routine keep your legs straight and your knees locked. This movement is recommended for those with spondylolysis or spondylolisthesis.

### Walking

As Thoreau said, "Simplify, simplify." Walking is a simple activity that is consistently touted as the best form of exercise because it utilizes so much of the body and helps improve the cardiopulmonary system. When you walk briskly with arms swinging and head held high, your midsection (trunk) rotates and gently stretches the fibers in the disks, which keeps them nourished and flexible. Walking is fun (walk with a friend or take a Walkman if you want) and affordable—but do invest in a good pair of walking shoes. A brisk thirty-minute walk five times a week provides good aerobic conditioning and strengthens the back. If you are just starting to heal from your back-pain episode, you will need to build up to this amount gradually.

When walking, remember the following tips:

- Be aware of your posture. Your abdominal muscles should hold your lower back in alignment.
- Walk with enthusiasm. Swing your arms and allow your hips and legs to stride pointing forward.
- Avoid bouncing or moving excessively from side to side. This places strain on your back and hips.
- Don't be upset if you are not able to walk briskly. Research at the Cooper Institute for Aerobics Research in Dallas shows that even a slow, even pace helps the heart and lowers cholesterol levels.
- Walking up and down hills places strain on the lower back.

If the weather is a problem, find an enclosed mall and walk through it several times. Many malls have programs that allow "walking club" members to come in and walk before the facility opens. Contact the management of your local mall for information.

### Bicycling

Bicycling, either on the road or on a stationary bike, is another aerobic option, depending on the seat type and height and how you position your hands and neck. Choose a comfortable seat: The small, hard racing seats found on many outdoor and stationary bikes are bothersome to many people. You may want to switch to a broad saddle or padded model. The seat height should allow you to reach the pedals comfortably without stretching out your legs. Your back should be straight; avoid the forward lean on the handlebars that places the back into a C-curve.

### Other Sports

Other sports, such as tennis (quick turns and motions), jogging (high impact), bowling (twisting, weight released far from body), weight lifting (strains, pulls, etc.), or golf (forward bending, twisting) may be your passion. Such activities should be avoided until your back is prepared for the added stresses these activities bring. Depending on the type of back injury and how well you strengthen your back and abdominal muscles, you can probably return to these sports if you take the necessary precautions.

# MYOTHERAPY

Myotherapy (*myo* = "muscle"; also called trigger-point myotherapy) is a hands-on treatment based on the concept that applying pressure to *trigger points*—spots in the muscles that have been injured or irritated in some way—can significantly reduce or eliminate pain. Pressure is applied using the fingers, knuckles, and elbows. Trigger points are caused by falls, strains, sprains, bumps, or any other incidents you may or may not remember. Myotherapists say that most people acquired their first trigger points as they came down the birth canal and have been accumulating more ever since.

According to Bonnie Prudden, a myotherapist and director of the Institute for Physical Fitness and Myotherapy in

Arizona, back pain is caused by a combination of three conditions: chronic muscle deficiency caused by lack of exercise; chronic strain caused by poor muscle strength and tone; and chronic pain due to trigger points that cause weak muscles to spasm. Diet and exercise are the recommended treatments for all three conditions, with the addition of myotherapy for the third. Prudden maintains that 95 percent of chronic pain can be reversed using myotherapy, good nutrition, and a sound movement program.

## Myotherapy and Your Back Pain

The number-one condition for which people seek myotherapy is back pain, especially lower back pain. Fortunately myotherapists report an 80 to 90 percent success rate treating this condition. If you have a friend or partner who would like to do a simple treatment on you, we provide some guidelines below. We recommend, however, that you experience at least one professional treatment so that you will understand what to expect during a session and so that you can ask questions.

Here are two easy treatments for lower back pain. Treatments are done while you lie on your stomach on a firm, comfortable surface, such as a padded mat or futon. You may want to wear a swimsuit or body suit so that your partner can mark the trigger points once he or she has located them. This can be done using a washable marker or small sticky labels that can be removed easily. The instructions below are addressed to your partner.

### *Lower-Back Treatment A*

1. Refer to points A, B, and C in Figure II-16. Place your elbow on one of the spots and slowly apply pressure at an angle—DO NOT apply pressure straight down. Trigger points can be very painful. If your

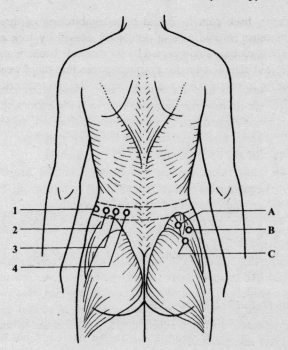

**II-16  Myotherapy pressure points for lower back pain**

"patient" responds by flinching, trying to leap off the table, or another obvious response, you have found a trigger point. Place your free hand flat on the area next to or around the trigger point. As you maintain pressure on the trigger point for seven seconds, also press down with your other hand. The second hand diffuses some of the pain caused when the trigger point is treated.

2. Mark the point so that you will know you have already treated that spot.

3. If your patient does not respond to the first spot you pressed, move your elbow around in the same area

and try again, maintaining the same amount of pressure. Once you find the other two spots, repeat the process above for each.

4. Now that you have released some of the spasm, you need to help the muscle relax. Have your friend *slowly* roll over onto one side with the buttock that was treated being up. You may or may not need to assist your friend with the following stretches.

4a. Slowly bend the top knee up to the chest.

4b. Now extend the leg straight down until it is about eight inches above the leg that is resting on the ground. The toes should *not* be pointed.

4c. Lower the raised leg and rest it on the bottom leg.

5. Repeat 4a–c four times.

6. Repeat the sequence 1–4c for the other side of the body.

### Lower-Back Treatment B

1. As your friend is lying facedown on the table, imagine he or she is wearing a belt that has eight notches across the back. These notches represent possible trigger points (see Figure II-16) and are labeled 1, 2, 3, and 4 on each side of the spine. Stand or kneel on the side farthest away from the number 2 of the side you are currently treating. Place your elbow against point 2, press down, and pull toward you, as if you wanted to get under the bulging muscles you are pressing. Hold this point (and all subsequent points) for seven seconds.

2. Next treat spot 1 by pressing down and outward.

3. Move your elbow about one inch horizontally out past spot 2 to spot 3. Press down and pull toward you.

4. Spot 4 is just above the bony rim of the pelvis and just below the rib cage. Reach across the back and approx-

imately halfway down your friend's side. Place your elbow and pull toward you and up.

5. To stretch out the muscles you just treated, ask your friend to get up on hands and knees and arch the back up like a cat ready to attack. The head should drop down and the elbows should remain locked.

6. While keeping the arms locked, the back should drop down like that of a horse with a saddle on. The head should be brought up.

7. Repeat steps 5 and 6 four times.

8. Have your friend lie down again and repeat the entire sequence (steps 1–7) on the other side of the spine.

## What Should I Expect from a Myotherapist?

Because *myotherapy* is a generic term for muscle therapy, some bodywork therapists claim to be myotherapists. If you want to see a *certified* trigger-point myotherapist, however—one who has been trained at a school for myotherapists—you must get a referral by a physician. Certified myotherapists will not treat you unless you have one. See Appendix A for information on myotherapists.

Once you arrive at the myotherapist's office with your referral and information about your condition, you and the practitioner will discuss the treatment. Then, according to his or her tools of the trade, the therapist will follow the general procedure described in the self-myotherapy instructions above: find a trigger point, apply pressure for seven seconds, and move on to the next point. Professional treatments are much more thorough than self-therapy, and the therapists know just how much pressure to apply.

A session typically lasts ninety minutes, and for several days afterward you will probably experience a slight soreness and a feeling like your muscles want to return to their old tense position. Each subsequent treatment will further train your muscles to remain in their proper position, and the exercises the myotherapist will recommend you do between sessions will help in this regard as well. How many sessions will you need? Each case differs, but most myotherapists say five to eight treatments usually provide the relief people want.

## How Does Myotherapy Work?

Many conventional and holistic practitioners recommend myotherapy for pain relief because it works. How it works remains to be determined. Myotherapists believe that trigger points lie in wait until something sets them off, such as overexertion, sleeping in an awkward position, a fall or automobile accident, or stress. The resultant pain may occur at a trigger point or at another location where the trigger point "refers" the pain. Myotherapists have mapped these referral sites and so know which areas on the body to treat for back pain. After any myotherapy treatment, stretching and movement are necessary to keep the muscles limber.

Bonnie Prudden, who started the institute after she studied with myotherapy pioneer Dr. Janet Travell and two other innovators in the field—Drs. Hans Kraus and Desmond Tivy—once asked Dr. Travell why myotherapy works. Travell replied, "You are denying the trigger point oxygen." Myotherapy, then, "chokes" the life out of trigger points and helps put a little life back into your back!

## OSTEOPATHY

When Juanita hurt her back while moving furniture one weekend, she made an appointment to see her family osteopath for a manipulation. Victor called his osteopath two days after he injured his back during a touch football game and a coughing spell sent sharp pains through his back. Why do Juanita and Victor and many other people seek care for their back from an osteopath? One reason is that osteopathic manipulation is very effective for many people with back pain. We explain below.

Osteopathy is one of two schools of Western medicine— the other is conventional, or allopathic, medicine. While conventional doctors focus on a specific complaint, such as a strained lower back or neck pain, osteopaths pay attention to all parts of the body and how any of them are affected by or have an impact on the primary complaint. During their osteopathic training they learn manipulative skills, and some use this hands-on therapy as the primary focus in their practice. *Osteopathy* literally means "bone disease," but the founder of osteopathy, Dr. Andrew Taylor Still, used the word to describe the relationship between a disorder and a misalignment of the bones. Osteopaths manipulate the spine to correct conditions that interfere with nervous activity or blood flow and cause pain, numbness, weakness, and other symptoms.

Both M.D.s and D.O.s (doctors of osteopathy) go through similar training up through the postgraduate level. After that point the focus shifts considerably for those who enter osteopathic school. Osteopaths receive comprehensive medical instruction that has a holistic, hands-on approach. They are taught to consider the entire body and how it functions as a whole when examining a patient. This approach is taken because osteopathy is based on the concepts that the human body and its functions, mind, and spirit are interdependent; that the body naturally seeks self-healing and self-regulation when faced with disease; and that health depends on an unobstructed flow of circulatory, neural, and nutritional energy throughout the body.

Osteopaths also study emotional and psychological factors and their influence on the body. Many osteopaths later incorporate homeopathy, acupuncture, massage, and other holistic therapies into their practices as well.

## Osteopathic Manipulation and Your Back Pain

The body has several mechanisms that act as shock absorbers. These include the lumbar, cervical, and thoracic vertebrae; and the hip, knee, ankle, arch, and sacrum. An injury or disturbance to any of these areas can throw the body out of balance and cause, among other things, back pain. When you make your first visit to an osteopath, you will discuss your medical history, including the incident you know or believe caused your back pain, plus any falls or accidents experienced since childhood. Along with questions about family background, previous and current medical conditions, and medication use will be lifestyle questions such as type of job, amount and kinds of stress, sleep patterns, social activities, details about food intake, and use of alcohol, tobacco, or drugs.

The medical evaluation typically includes a neurologic, orthopedic, and psychiatric examination. The osteopath will palpate (examine by touch) your spine and related structures to locate any tender points and to evaluate your posture. The alignment of your spine will be checked while you are both seated and lying down, both faceup and facedown. You may be asked to bend forward and to the sides, to lift your knees, and do other simple movements, which help the practitioner determine whether your pelvis and the base of your spine are balanced and symmetrical (see Figure II-17). Once the examination is complete, the osteopath may take X rays to rule out any physical disorder if something during the evaluation raised suspicions. Generally, however, osteopaths order radiographs and other studies only when absolutely necessary.

## CHOOSING A PHYSICIAN/HOLISTIC PRACTITIONER

You've visited a new physician or holistic practitioner for the first time and you need to decide whether you want to continue to see this individual. Here are some questions you can ask yourself to help you make a final decision:

- Was your appointment time honored?
- Is the office adequately accessible to you in terms of neighborhood, parking, distance?
- Does the physician appear to personally represent an unhealthy lifestyle; that is, smoking, overweight, stressed, drinking, fatigue?
- Is the office environment relaxed and pleasant? Is the support staff helpful and friendly?
- Did the physician take adequate time to listen to your concerns and fears and seem genuinely interested in what you had to say?
- Did the physician fully diagnose and/or discuss your condition with you?
- Did the physician order expensive tests or urge you to undergo testing you believe is unnecessary?
- Did the practitioner prescribe medications you are not confident in taking because you received little or no information about them or they have known adverse effects?
- Do you have confidence in the therapy or treatment the physician recommended for you?
- Do you feel the physician allowed you adequate time to make decisions about treatment, or do you feel you were pressured?

- Overall, how did you feel about the experience?
  (Adapted from the American Holistic Medical Association recommendations)

Nearly everyone gets some relief at their first visit. The
exact type of manipulation you receive will depend on the
osteopath's findings. An example of a manipulation for
lower back pain is shown in Figure II-18. You will also be
expected to take much of the responsibility for your recovery. As the osteopath uses manipulation to remove the ob-
structions to health, he or she may also recommend specific
exercises, relaxation techniques, dietary modifications, or
psychological consultation; you may get a prescription for
pain medication, a homeopathic or botanical remedy, or a
referral to a physical therapist. In other words the approach
to treatment of your back pain is a holistic one.

## How Does Osteopathy Work?

Osteopaths conduct an extensive examination in order to
identify the cause of your pain, including the possibility of
other medical problems. Once the cause or probable cause
has been determined, your osteopathic treatment will be
unique. Much of the success of the treatment depends on
the ability of the osteopath to locate the specific areas of the
spine or other parts of the body that need adjustment and on
how the manipulation is done. Your part is to help the manipulation "stick" by making the lifestyle adjustments the
practitioner recommends.

During a typical session the practitioner performs only
the manipulations you need. Osteopaths focus not so much
on structure (as chiropractors do) as they do on functional
ability. If the limb or joint moves well and does not hinder
full function, the area may not need aggressive treatment.

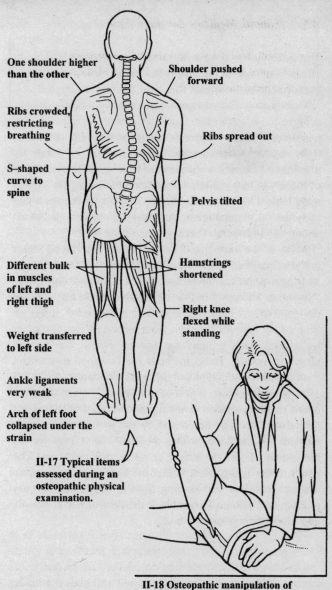

One shoulder higher than the other

Shoulder pushed forward

Ribs crowded, restricting breathing

Ribs spread out

S–shaped curve to spine

Pelvis tilted

Different bulk in muscles of left and right thigh

Hamstrings shortened

Weight transferred to left side

Right knee flexed while standing

Ankle ligaments very weak

Arch of left foot collapsed under the strain

II-17 Typical items assessed during an osteopathic physical examination.

II-18 Osteopathic manipulation of lower thoracic vertebrae

The goals are to treat with minimum force for maximum effect and to use as few treatments as necessary so as not to overstretch the ligaments that hold the bones together.

Osteopaths use various manipulative techniques to achieve these goals: the gentle hold of tense muscles in a positional release known as counterstrain; the stretch of tight muscles using muscle energy; and short, rapid replacement of bones when they are misaligned are just three of those you may experience while on the osteopath's treatment table. Others include various myofascial therapies and craniosacral manipulation, the latter of which is discussed under "Craniosacral Therapy" (see page 99).

Many of the more than 33,500 D.O.s in the United States are also qualified to give specialized injection therapy such as trigger-point treatment and ligament strengthening (see "Injection Therapy" in Part III). Both of these methods are designed to provide rapid, long-lasting pain relief, although they do not cure the problem. Your osteopath may use other techniques, such as massage and movement, to increase range of motion. These methods are designed to improve joint mobility and alignment, increase circulation, and stimulate body functions. If you hear a "crack" when the osteopath makes a sudden thrust manipulation, don't jump off the table. This may be caused by the movement of small menisci, or cartilage, within the joint, or it may be the movement of air; the actual cause is still unknown. The result of the realignment is that the bones no longer press against nerves or surrounding tissues, which can be very painful, and also no longer block the flow of nerve, lymph, and blood throughout the body.

# PHYSICAL DEVICES

Braces and corsets, two of the most common physical devices orthopedists prescribe, are useful for some people who need abdominal support, posture correction, reduced pressure on the disks, or restriction of certain movements during the healing process. Some people prefer to use these physical aids because they are psychologically as well as physically comforting during a bout of back pain, helping them to feel more secure. On the down side, long-term or incorrect use of physical devices can cause abdominal or other muscles to become weak. When unbraced muscles overcompensate for the immobilized ones, this can lead to an imbalance of muscle strength and flexibility. That's why these devices should be used as short-term solutions only.

Braces and corsets are usually worn under clothing and come in various forms. Braces have metal stays and are sturdier than corsets, and they lack flexibility. Corsets are made of elastic, fit close to the body, and can be adjusted. In most cases both braces and corsets are worn only until individuals have healed enough to start an active movement routine. People who engage in lifting as part of their job often continue to use an external corset as needed; many grocery store clerks, for example, now wear them to prevent back stress and injury.

Back disorders that may require use of a brace or corset for longer periods of time include scoliosis and spondylolisthesis. These devices are designed to decrease swayback, reinforce weak abdominal muscles, and limit the amount of motion. Elderly individuals who are unable to exercise because of a compression fracture or degenerative disease may also benefit from a brace.

# POLARITY THERAPY

Have you ever thought of your body as being like a battery, with positive and negative charges? According to Dr. Randolph Stone, an osteopath, chiropractor, naturopath, and founder of polarity therapy, the head and upper body are positive while the feet and lower body are negative. He and those who practice polarity therapy believe the life force constantly flows through these two extreme points along five predictable pathways, similar to the meridian concept (see Figure II-19).

Polarity therapy is the culmination of therapeutic techniques Dr. Stone studied around the world and represents what he believes are the best: reflexology, deep massage, Ayurvedic medicine, and craniosacral therapy. It is based on the idea that pain is the result of blocked or sluggish energy. Dr. Stone determined that the five energy centers in the body must be in balance in order for the life force to flow smoothly.

Polarity therapists typically use a three-part holistic approach to treatment: bodywork (manipulation), stretching exercises, and nutrition. While it's true that bodywork alone will probably give you significant relief, the incorporation of stretching and a healthy diet is more likely to provide complete, lasting relief.

## Polarity Therapy for Your Backache

The goal of polarity therapists is to help you, through the experience of bodywork, understand your body and how it operates so that you can care for yourself. Polarity is both a preventive and a treatment tool for back pain.

Professional polarity therapists use three types of manipulations to release blocked energy:

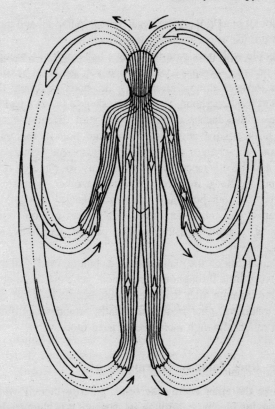

**II-19** Life energy circulating through the energy channels. Each energy current has a charge and flows from the body through a particular toe or finger

- *Neutral:* light touches with the fingertips which soothe and balance the energy
- *Positive:* application of light to medium pressure with the hands, which is meant to move blocked energy
- *Negative:* deep massage and pressure into the tissues, which can be painful

Not all practitioners use negative manipulation, and those who do, use it occasionally and selectively.

People with back pain make up a large part of the clientele polarity therapists treat. When you go for a session, wear loose clothing and expect a full-body treatment that lasts at least one hour. You will be asked to lie on a padded table—either faceup or facedown to start. Because everyone has a positive and a negative charge, polarity therapists channel the charges through their hands—one being positive and the other negative—to stimulate your energy flow. As energy flows from one hand to the other, it creates a current on your body and moves your energy along. Your therapist will move her hands to all areas of your body, pausing to apply pressure, grasp a part of your body, and move energy.

Depending on the manipulation technique used, you may feel very little throughout the session, yet experience complete relaxation after it is over. Some people doze off during treatment. One treatment usually provides significant pain relief, although most people need more.

## How Does Polarity Therapy Work?

Like the other energy therapies, polarity therapy works by moving bioenergy through areas where it is blocked. It is most effective in relieving pain if you embrace all three of its elements, which work together to stimulate and maintain bioenergy flow, rid the body of toxins, and restore harmony between your positive and negative poles. There are more than 130 certified practitioners in the United States.

# REFLEXOLOGY

You may have seen foot and hand charts on which there are so many lines and dots that the foot and hand look like maps of strange continents with dozens of cities named after body parts. These are maps of the reflex sites on your feet, hands, and even ears that, when pressed and held, can gradually relieve the pain, tenderness, or other imbalance in the area that corresponds to that body site.

If reflexology sounds similar to acupressure, you are right: The points used in both treatments are alike. In acupressure the points relate to specific body locations by means of the meridians; in reflexology the points correspond to nerve endings via nerve pathways. When you press on a reflex point and experience soreness, it usually means there are crystallized calcium and acid deposits on the nerve endings. As you continue to apply gradual pressure to a spot that corresponds to your back, you stimulate that point, which then prompts the nerves to energize the related area of your back. The gradual pressure breaks up and dissolves the accumulated deposits. You are the best judge of how much pressure feels good yet is firm enough to stimulate the point. This makes reflexology an excellent self-treatment for back pain.

## Reflexology for Your Back Pain

Use reflexology to relieve your back pain by referring to figure II-20–22 and by following the guidelines below. If the spots you press on your foot, hand, or ear are very tender, try gradual, prolonged light pressure until the deposits begin to dissolve and you are comfortable applying more pressure.

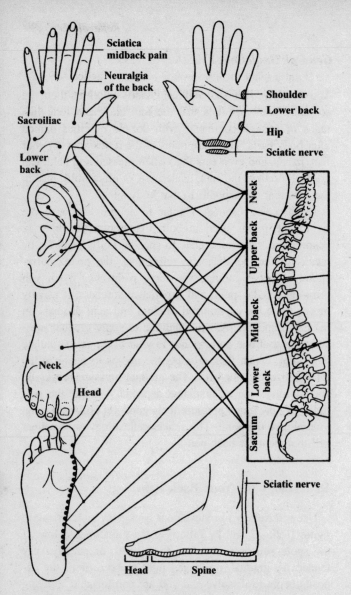

Sciatica
midback pain

Neuralgia
of the back

Sacroiliac

Lower
back

Shoulder
Lower back
Hip
Sciatic nerve

Neck

Upper back

Mid back

Lower back

Sacrum

Neck

Head

Sciatic nerve

Head        Spine

II-20–22

## General Guidelines

- Find a quiet location where you can practice reflexology uninterrupted for ten to fifteen minutes.
- When you find a tender reflex point, focus on it and note how you feel as you apply pressure. You may want to close your eyes to help you concentrate. Hold the tender spot until the soreness decreases.
- If your fingernails are not short enough to do reflexology comfortably, use the eraser end of a pencil to apply pressure.
- Not all reflex points are the same size; some are no bigger than the head of a pin, while others are slightly larger than pea-sized. You will become familiar with them with practice.
- Different reflexology charts often vary somewhat in terms of which points correspond to which organs and body sites. Explore your own feet and rub any painful or tender spot until the pain decreases. Note the effect this has on your back pain. Tender points may be sore because they correspond to a completely different problem. Holistically speaking, however, all body parts are interrelated and impact the whole, so any sensitive reflex points you treat will have some effect on your back pain.

## Foot Reflexology

Begin each session with an overall foot massage. Use a light, greaseless lotion or herbal oil. (See Figure II-20–22 for specific pressure areas.)

- Grasp the heel, toes, or ankle of your left foot with your left hand and place the thumb of your right hand on the sole of your foot at the heel. Keep your thumb slightly bent at the joint as you apply steady, even pressure to the sole of your foot. Move toward the toes using a kneading action: press a spot, release, move toward the toes slightly, press again, and so on. Once you reach your toes, return to your heel and start from a new spot. After you have massaged the entire bottom of your foot, do a similar massage to the top of the foot. (If you have limited time, skip this part.) If you have time, repeat the entire massage. If not, allow time to do the sequence on the other foot.

- After you finish the massage, go back and focus on any spots that were tender. Hold these points until the pain subsides. These may correspond to areas of back pain.
- Walking barefoot on sand, grass, or unobstructed earth is an excellent natural way to stimulate the reflex points on your feet. If you are a ''tender foot,'' start with sand or grass.

### Hand Reflexology

The reflex points along your thumb and index finger correspond to the back and neck (see Figure II-20–22). If you have lower back pain, you may discover a tender spot in the webbing between your thumb and index finger. Experiment with this area.

Once you find a sensitive spot on your hand, hold it for several minutes until you can feel a steady pulse beneath your finger. Continue to apply pressure until the pulse is strong and balanced, which indicates that the blockage has been broken up and circulation has improved.

### Ear Reflexology

When working on the ears, the right ear corresponds to the right side of the back; the left ear corresponds to the left side of the back. If your pain is located on the spine or center of your back, work on both ears. Apply pressure to each tender spot until the pain lessens and the spot feels warm or pulsates (see Figure II-20–22).

## How Does Reflexology Work?

In theory reflexology is similar to acupressure and acupuncture in that all of these systems explain that their benefits are the result of endorphin release. Those who practice reflexology believe it opens up the lymph system and allows the healing power of the lymphatic fluids to bathe injured and painful areas. When you work all the reflex points on your feet, you are in essence doing a complete body massage. Thus you send healing energy to your entire body, not just your back.

As with any form of bodywork, stop treatment on a very sore spot after you have applied some brief, gentle pressure there, and then return to it after you have opened up other blocked areas. You may need to repeat treatments several times, especially if you have chronic pain. Don't get discouraged. It takes the body some time to adjust to reflexology and other forms of bodywork—but it is worth it.

## TAI CHI

*When the lowest vertebrae are plumb erect,*
*The spirit reaches to the top of the head.*
*With the top of the head as if suspended from above;*
*The whole body feels itself light and nimble.*
*—The Classics of Tai-Chi-Ch'uan*

The art of tai chi chuan (tai chi) is viewed in several different ways by Westerners. It's been called slow-motion calisthenics, moving meditation, or poetry in motion. Other people point out its many health benefits, for both body and mind; some immediately think of martial arts.

Tai chi is all of these things and more. It brings together the Chinese philosophy of yang (positive) and yin (negative), the eternal opposites. In tai chi, people move from yin to yang (from soft, slow rest to hard, fast motion) and vice versa in harmonious balance. The result, say the Chinese, is a discipline that is not too fast, not too slow, not too hard, and not too soft in execution.

Because tai chi is practiced in slow motion, some people say it is "easy" and could not possibly build strength, stamina, or flexibility. Quite the contrary. Tai chi practitioners explain that slow movement is difficult and that as tai chi students develop greater slowness, they increase their ability for greater speed. In tai chi a primary goal is alert relaxation, and with it comes improved flexibility. In addition, moving in controlled slow motion also builds muscle strength and endurance. In short it has all the makings of a great back-pain therapy.

## Tai Chi for Your Back Pain

The recommended way to learn tai chi is to take a course. Many health or community centers, hospitals, and schools either sponsor or offer tai chi classes, for beginners to advanced students. Classes at each ability level usually last six to eight weeks, after which you can move to the next level if you wish.

When you choose a tai chi class, ask about the approach or philosophy of the instructor. Some teachers focus on the physical health benefits while others emphasize the calm, relaxed nature of the art. The ideal teacher for people with back pain is one who combines both. Naturally those who focus on the martial arts aspect need to be avoided at this stage.

From your very first tai chi lesson, you will train both your body and your mind. Often instructors offer colorful imagery to help students understand the mental part of tai chi at the same time that they learn the physical movements. You may hear suggestions like "move like a lion" and "push away as if you are moving the wind"; these are meant to help you visualize and experience tai chi. This experience includes learning how to relax all of your major muscles and to move without stress and tension, as well as achieve inner calm, awareness, and peace.

Before beginning tai chi, consult with your doctor. Tell your tai chi instructor about the extent of your back problem. Then dress for success: Wear light, loose clothing— sweat clothes are good—and tennis or aerobic shoes. Avoid heels or shoes with hard soles.

Traditional tai chi includes more than one hundred movements. Many modified forms have been created over the centuries, however, and today abbreviated versions usually have twenty-four to forty-eight positions—plenty for our purposes.

Below are two warm-up movements and the first two tai chi movements to give you a feel for this ancient art form. When you reach the end of tai chi movement 2, you will be standing with your arms stretched out diagonal to your body. We leave you there, poised and ready to explore more tai chi on your own!

### Warm-up 1 *(see Figure II-23)*
- Stand straight with your feet together and your knees straight but not locked. Place your hands on your waist with your fingers pointed toward the small of your back and your thumbs forward.
- Push your stomach forward with your fingers.
- Rotate your waist thirty-two times to the right and thirty-two times to the left.

This warm-up strengthens the waist and stomach muscles.

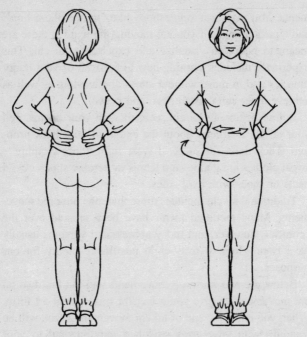

**II-23   Tai chi warm-up exercise: waist/stomach-rotating exercise**

### *Warm-up 2 (see Figure II-24)*

- Stand straight with your feet parallel and about one foot apart.
- Place your hands at the sides of your lower hips. Your thumbs should face forward while your fingers point back and down.
- With your left hand push your hip toward the right and rotate your hips in an oval pattern thirty-two times to the right and thirty-two times to the left.

This warm-up loosens the hip joints.

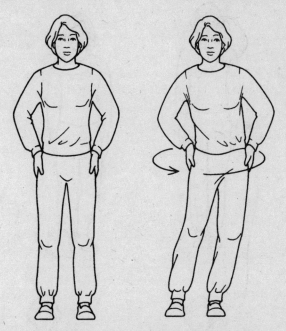

**II-24   Tai chi warm-up exercise: hip-rotating exercise**

## *Movement 1: Strike Palm to Ask Buddha (see Figure II-25)*

- Stand straight, feet together and hands at your sides.
- Turn your right foot outward 45 degrees.
- Bend both knees, then extend your left foot forward about two feet. Keep the left knee straight, your heel on the ground, and your toes up.
- Raise both arms to shoulder level and face palms forward.
- While keeping your arms up, bring your hands together until they almost touch. Your hands should be about eighteen inches from your chest.

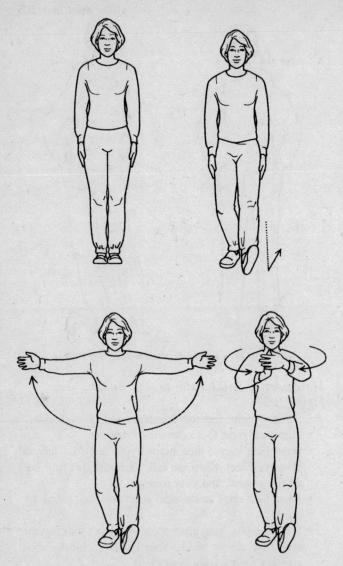

**II-25  Tai chi movement: strike palm to ask Buddha**

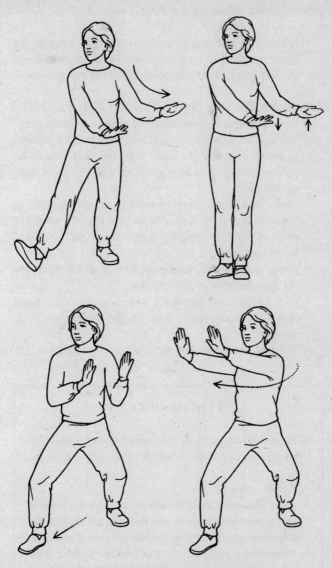

II-26  Tai chi movement: grasp bird's tail

- Keeping your hands open, bend the right hand at the wrist so that it is now perpendicular to the middle of the left hand. Hold this position for several seconds.

## Movement 2: Grasp Bird's Tail *(see Figure II-26)*

- From the ending position of movement 1, move your left foot back past your right heel until it is 45 degrees in back of your right foot. Your left foot should be perpendicular to your right foot and the right toes should point up.
- Move your hands down to waist level and diagonal to your left hip. Keep both elbows bent slightly, your left palm up and the right palm down. Your right leg should be straight and the toes up.
- Bring your right leg back until the ball of the right foot touches the arch of the left foot.
- Step forward and diagonally with your right foot. Bend both knees and center your weight. Keep your back straight.
- Twist at the waist and shoulder until your hands are even.

---

### TAI CHI PRACTICE TIPS

- Be patient with yourself. The movements and positions in tai chi are likely different from those you have done in the past.
- Practice every day.
- Every movement must include the entire body. It takes time to remember to move your right and left hands at the same time or to move your legs and arms simultaneously.
- When first learning tai chi, it is common to have difficulty matching the movements with the breathing. Concentrate. Movements should be even and flowing and in

harmony with your breathing. This, too, will come with practice.

- Many positions require that you stand on a "hollow" or a "solid" leg. A "solid" leg is one that is bent and supports your entire weight, while the "hollow" leg bears no weight and is thus free to move.

## How Does Tai Chi Work for Back Pain?

Tai chi is a gentle movement therapy in which every move is natural—the way nature designed the body to move. When the postures, or positions, are done correctly, the spinal column moves into natural alignment. This in turn keeps the internal organs in their proper place and prevents them from causing unnatural pressure internally, which is a cause of back pain.

Tai chi is also good for bones. According to tai chi tenets, the vital energy of those who practice the art accumulates just below the navel in the hara (see page 90). Gradually it becomes hot and travels throughout the body, clearing out blocked energy and opening up joints. The bones themselves become stronger because the vital energy condenses inside the bones and forms extra marrow.

Controlled slow motion builds strength, and strong muscles are much less likely to cause back pain. Another benefit, of course, is the feeling of inner peace that moves in as stress and tension move out.

# THERAPEUTIC TOUCH

*Nature alone cures. . . . And what nursing has to do . . . is to put the patient in the best condition for nature to act upon him.*

—*Florence Nightingale*

Therapeutic touch is a timeless healing art that is derived from the laying on of hands. We have elsewhere introduced the idea of the vital force—the energy that flows within you—and how you can release and manipulate it. Therapeutic touch involves manipulation of the energy that extends beyond the body, like a force field. It is being used in conventional hospitals and is an accepted clinical therapeutic practice all over the United States for conditions ranging from headache to infections to asthma to back pain. It has been taught to more than thirty-seven thousand nurses, doctors, and health practitioners and is used every day in hospitals around the world.

Therapeutic touch got its start in this country in New York City hospitals by a therapist named Dona Kunz. In the mid 1970s Dr. Dolores Krieger, Ph.D., helped her develop the method and gave it the name it has today. (Read about the development of therapeutic touch in Krieger's book; see "Suggestions for Further Reading.")

Therapeutic touch complements medical and surgical procedures; it does not replace them. It can be done by anyone who is willing to learn the techniques and who possesses the following qualities: (a) good health—a general feeling of well-being and a sense of wholeness; (b) compassion—the ability to empathize with individuals who need treatment and an unselfish desire to help; (c) self-discipline—required because therapeutic touch must be practiced regularly; and (d) confidence, based on experience and knowledge, that therapeutic touch is effective. This last quality takes time to develop and will grow as you practice.

## Therapeutic Touch for Your Back Pain

Therapeutic touch can be done by a trained therapist or a partner or friend who has learned the techniques. You and a friend may want to take a class in therapeutic touch so that you can treat each other. It is helpful to have a professional work with you and explain the sensations you will feel while you learn so that you will have a point of reference. The most common sensations are described in the box on page 213.

Practitioners of therapeutic touch generally follow a method, which is described below. Although we explain the method in steps as if they were separate, they are like streams that flow into each other and work together. As you practice the techniques, you will experience this interconnectedness. When you first visit a therapeutic touch practitioner or teacher, your experience will likely be similar to the one described here.

1. **Centering:** The practitioner must first quiet his or her mind and clear it of chatter and everyday thoughts. Often a short meditation or centering exercise brings this about. She may close her eyes, breathe deeply, and picture herself as energy or as receiving energy. Some practitioners focus on an image in nature or on light. Whatever technique works is okay. Your therapist may massage your shoulders and neck at this point as a way of helping both of you relax and of making a vital connection between the two of you.

2. **Assessment:** The assessment can be done in whatever position is most practical and comfortable for both you and the therapist. The most desirable position is

one that allows assessment of your entire energy field—that is, so that the therapist's hands can pass three to five inches, unhindered, from your skin surface over most or all of your body. Seated sideways on a chair with your back exposed allows a good assessment (see Figure II-27). During a typical assessment the therapist holds her hands with the palms toward you, one hand in front and the other in back, as she passes them down your body from head to toe. Then she kneels in front of you and passes both hands down the front and repeats the same for your back. The therapist notes subtle changes in temperature or any vibration in your energy field that indicates congestion or weakened energy flow, such as backache, infection, or a healed wound. The entire assessment takes about thirty seconds.

3. **Clearing Congestion:** To break up the blocked energy, the therapist makes repeated sweeping motions downward with her hands, which carry the energy out through your arms and legs. At the end of each sweep she shakes the energy off and sends it away. This clearing of congested energy is done for the entire body, even if the pain is concentrated only in the back, so that the energy can flow unobstructed throughout the body.

4. **Balancing the Energy Field:** As the therapist unblocks bottled-up energy, any gaps in your energy field fill up because your body inherently wants to be balanced and whole. As a finishing touch, the therapist does a final sweeping of your body's energy fields to smooth out the energy flow and fill in any holes in the field.

---

**ASSESSMENT SENSATIONS**

Whoever performs the assessment will feel the energy flowing, either freely or with "stops and starts." Changes in energy flow are difficult to describe in words, yet that's all we have. The therapist (or your partner/friend, or yourself if you are doing a treatment on someone) may sense the following cues from the energy field, which have the following indications:

- Heat, heaviness, pressure, or thickness indicates loose congestion
- Coldness, lack of movement, emptiness indicate obstruction or tight congestion
- Coolness or a decrease in the energy's rhythm indicates partially obstructed area
- Pulling or tugging sensation indicates a deficit
- Pins and needles, static, disordered vibrations indicate a local imbalance

(Adapted from Janet Macrae, *Therapeutic Touch: A Practical Guide*)

---

## How Does Therapeutic Touch Work?

As one woman said after undergoing several therapeutic touch sessions for chronic lower back pain, "Do we have to know 'why' for everything? Sometimes we just need to accept things." Although therapeutic touch has its skeptics, many individuals who experience it say it leaves them remarkably relaxed and feeling much less or no pain. Therapeutic-touch practitioners believe that life energy flows

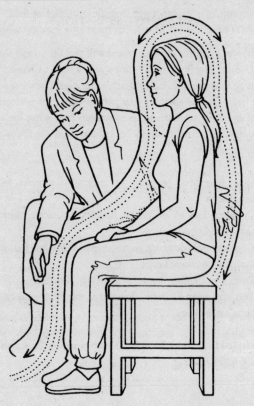

**II-27  Assessment of an individual's energy field during therapeutic touch**

from their hands into the energy field of their clients. Once the clients receive that energy, they internalize it and allow it to balance their own weak field. A balanced energy field allows the body to heal itself. And therapeutic touch has withstood the scrutiny of scientific investigation. Acute pain responds more quickly to therapeutic touch than does chronic pain. If you don't get significant relief at first, don't give up! There are no ill effects from connecting with and balancing your energy.

# THERMOTHERAPY

*Thermo-* ("heat") therapy relaxes tense muscles and increases circulation and the metabolic rate. Application of heat before a movement routine can ease pain, warm the muscles, reduce spasm, and increase mobility.

Heat is not for everyone nor for all back pain, however, and it should be used with caution. A general rule is: No heat during the first twenty-four hours after injury. Applying heat too soon can increase swelling. But what about after that? Should you use heat or cold? Generally cold gives better relief for chronic low back pain, whereas heat is better in acute cases of pain. If the area you want to treat is swollen, do not apply heat. Excessive heat or heat applied for even a few minutes can cause skin damage; therefore avoid using heat if you have decreased sensation or impaired circulation. Some elderly people are very sensitive to heat, so thermotherapy is best avoided.

## Thermotherapy for Your Back Pain

Thermotherapy can be applied as either superficial or deep heat. *Superficial heat* includes heating pads, hot towels, whirlpools (see "Hydrotherapy"), and infrared light. This type of heat penetrates to the subcutaneous tissues—the top layers of the skin. To prevent burns, any heated item applied directly to the skin should be no greater than 100 degrees F and stay on the skin no longer than thirty minutes. If you use a heating pad, place it on top of the painful area. Avoid lying on a heating pad or sleeping with it on. If possible, use moist heat (hot, wet towels or hydrocollator packs) instead of a heating pad because the pad generates dry heat, which can dehydrate the treated area. Hydrocollator packs (also called gel packs, they are silica-gel-filled cotton bags you heat in hot water) can be heated to about 135 degrees F (use a candy or meat thermometer to check), but these should be wrapped in two towels before applying them to the back. These packs retain heat for a long time.

Infrared heating involves placing an infrared bulb above the painful area for twenty to thirty minutes. This method is effective for small areas and allows the therapist to closely monitor the site as it is treated.

*Deep heat* treatments reach to the bone, muscle, and ligaments. The two most common types are diathermy and ultrasound. *Diathermy* uses shortwave or microwave to deliver heat to deep structures and decrease pain. *Ultrasound* involves very low, subaudible sound waves that penetrate deeper than diathermy. These waves massage and heat tissue and muscle deep below the skin. Ultrasound provides only temporary pain relief and so must be repeated. A typical treatment routine includes a twenty-minute session three times a week for two to three weeks. It is not used for acute back pain, as the heat causes additional swelling to occur. Ultrasound must be done by a qualified therapist or practitioner and is usually part of an overall therapy program.

## TRACTION

Traction is the use of weights, pulleys, harnesses, or straps that pull the upper and lower parts of the body in opposite directions. Traction is an effective method for some individuals with neck or back pain. The amount of weight or other pressure used and the length of time a person is in traction depends on the individual and his or her condition.

Traction has been around since the days of Hippocrates, yet physicians still do not agree about how effective it is in treating low back pain, nor which variation should be used and when. Many doctors question whether traction is worth the time and effort, as there are many other therapies available for back pain. Most argue that it is not cost-effective to admit someone to the hospital for traction given the high cost of medical care. Others stress that its benefits appear to be short-lived. For these reasons traction, when used at all, is usually done on an outpatient basis, or patients rent or purchase traction devices designed for home use.

The basic idea behind traction is to stretch the muscles and ligaments and to relieve disk- or spinal-alignment problems, which it does by increasing the space between the vertebrae and enlarging the disk spaces. This action decreases intradiskal pressure and thus relieves pain. Traction comes in various forms, including the following:

- Light weights applied continuously for several hours
- Application of heavier weights for up to thirty minutes at a time
- Intermittent traction that is applied and released every few seconds
- Autotraction, in which individuals pull on a harness and regulate their own amount of traction (see Figure II-28)
- Manual-mechanical, often used by chiropractors, in which the individual is strapped to a specially designed divided table and pulled
- Gravity inversion, considered to be a form of autotraction by some health care professionals (see Figure II-29)

Traction on the lower back is used most often for a herniated nucleus pulposus—the jellylike center of the disk. The goal is to stretch the spine enough for the protruded disk to return to a normal or near-normal position.

Generally the results of studies in which one or more forms of traction have been analyzed and compared have not been promising, except for autotraction. Lewis shared his experience with autotraction, which he tried after spending nearly two years popping painkillers to control chronic back pain and muscle spasms that periodically kept him out of work for days at a time. After a visit to his physician he was referred to a physical therapist, who showed him how to use a home pelvic traction device in the therapist's office (see Figure II-29). Lewis liked the fact that he could control the amount of traction himself, and after using the device several times, bought one for home use. Two or three fifteen-minute sessions per day have significantly improved his pain and spasm. He now combines his traction sessions with a brief movement program and has not missed a day of work due to back pain in more than a year. When he skips several days, he notices the difference. This illustrates a point physicians often make, which is that traction provides short-term relief only. Once you stop, the vertebrae slowly return to their previous pain-producing positions.

*Gravity inversion* uses the body's weight rather than other physical weights to provide traction. Did you ever hang upside down on the monkey bars when you were a child? That was your first traction session. Now you are more sophisticated and place your feet in special boots that are attached to an overhead bar, strap yourself to a tilt table, or hook your legs around gravity-traction equipment. Studies show that gravity-inversion techniques can improve back pain and open up the lumbar spine up to 4.0 mm and relieve pressure on the disks. Some people do bent-knee

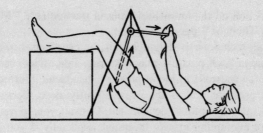

**II-28 Autotraction**

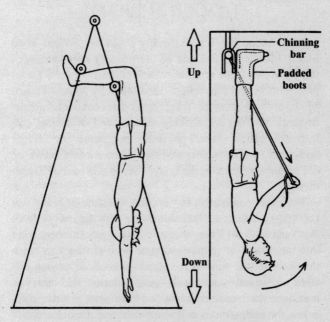

**II-29 Two types of gravity-inversion traction**

situps and other movements while in traction (see "Movement Therapy," page 164).

This technique is definitely not for everyone, however. Although back pressure may decrease, side effects can include an increase in blood pressure, headache, blurred vision, pressure behind the eyes, a stuffy nose, decreased heart rate, and retinal detachment. Consult your physician before attempting gravity inversion, especially if you have hypertension or glaucoma. For your own safety have someone with you when you do gravity inversion.

## TRAGER THERAPY

Another name for Trager therapy could be "When Mind Meets Muscle," since one of the primary components of this approach is the mind-to-muscle contact between Trager practitioners and their client. Developed by Milton Trager, M.D., in the 1920s, the Trager approach consists of gentle, rhythmic rocking and shaking motions and stretching, collectively called Psychophysical Integration or Trager bodywork, which is designed to subconsciously break up old tension patterns in the body. This is one part of Trager therapy.

The other component is "hookup," a state of being that Dr. Trager defines as "becoming one with the energy force that surrounds all living things." Trager practitioners enter this meditative or mind-meld state so that they can reach the unconscious mind of the client—where old tension patterns are stored—and convey new patterns. The theory is that once the mind sends the body the new, positive messages, the unconscious will remember, and the old negative patterns will be replaced by the new ones. While Trager practitioners work with a client, they are always asking themselves silently "What could be softer? What could be freer?" and communicating these thoughts to the unconscious mind and ultimately the muscles of their client. When you do Trager work on your own (see below), ask yourself these questions as well and communicate positive input into your unconscious.

## Trager Therapy and Your Back Pain

Back pain is one of the primary reasons people seek Trager therapy. A typical session with a Trager practitioner lasts sixty to ninety minutes, and during that time the therapist communicates with your muscles using gentle shaking and rocking actions and range-of-motion movements similar to massage strokes. The key to the session, however, is the mind-to-muscle contact between the practitioner and you. When there is synchronization between the mind of your therapist and your muscles, the movements you are put through release old neuromuscular tension and patterns. This release allows your energy and motions to flow freely, and pain is relieved. According to Trager, 90 percent of the clients with back pain that he has worked on have needed only one tablework session. He attributes this success rate to the practice of Mentastics, which is explained below.

## Trager Therapy On Your Own

To experience the benefits of Trager work at home, start with the "mental gymnastics" Dr. Trager developed to help keep the pain from his own congenital back problem, spondylolisthesis, under control. Called Trager Mentastics, they consist of simple, effortless dance movements that many say can make you feel as good as you would if you had done Trager sessions. The goal of Mentastics is hookup; the movements are based on expansion, not contraction, as many exercises are. Mentastics are taught to

Trager-therapy clients so that they can practice them at home and maintain the relaxed state they experience during a session.

If you incorporate Mentastics into your daily routine, you can ease current back pain and help prevent future occurrences. Try the sample Trager Mentastics explained below.

### *Mentastic 1*

Stand with your arms hanging loosely at your sides. Kick each leg once to each side so that you can see and feel your thigh muscles bounce. Do not let your foot touch the floor. The kick should be soft and light, not rough or done with anger. Feel the weight of your leg and the shaking in your calves and ankles. When you kick, it creates a jiggle in the lower back. Place your fingers on your lower back on the bony structure. Do you feel a bounce when you kick? If you do, this indicates a release of tension in the lower back. If you don't feel a bounce, do not try to make it bounce. Mentastics happen naturally, not with force.

Continue this Mentastic by walking along and pretending to kick a can or a stone. Take small steps and do not hold your foot out too long. The kick should be natural and rhythmic. If you feel pain, slow down. Every kick helps you develop more and more softness, which increases your hookup. Dr. Trager claims the Mentastic kick helps many people with chronic low back pain remain free from pain.

### *Mentastic 2*

This is an important Mentastic to improve your posture or, as Trager refers to it, develop elongation. Practice this Mentastic as you get up from and sit down in a chair and concentrate on your breathing. First, place a sturdy chair in a place where you have room to walk. Stand in front of the chair so that the backs of your legs touch the chair edge.

(The chair seat should be a little higher than the level of your knees.)

Exhale slowly and as you do, sit down. Allow the air to carry you to the seat. Once seated, lean forward slightly and inhale as you stand up, as if the air were making you rise. Repeat this sequence several times. The last time you rise, slowly raise your arms over your head and reach with your fingers to the sky. This is an elongated position. Do not stay there physically, but mentally picture yourself in this state. Allow your legs to dangle relaxed from your hips. Enjoy the feeling of elongation as tension drains from your back. Walk around the room for several minutes and repeat the sitting and elongation sequence. Practice this entire Mentastic several times a day.

## How Does the Trager Approach Work?

If you thought we were going to give you a definitive answer, we don't have one. Dr. Trager believes a key to the approach's success lies in the connection made with the mind. Once the unconscious mind is reached and a person is conveyed the feeling of being softer and lighter, old patterns can be released and with them pain and discomfort. He has successfully treated people with back pain, emphysema, and serious neuromuscular disorders such as muscular dystrophy, multiple sclerosis, and polio. In these latter diseases the Trager Approach has helped some individuals regain movement in limbs that were paralyzed. Dr. Trager posits that his approach allows the body to use muscle and nerve pathways left undamaged by the disease.

# VISUALIZATION AND GUIDED IMAGERY

*I am, as Protagoras says, the judge of the existence of the things that are to me and of the nonexistence of those that are not to me . . . man is the measure of all things.*

—*Socrates*

*Visualization* is a general term used to describe the use of various visual techniques to relax, reduce pain, and otherwise heal and treat disease. In visualization, people enter a very relaxed state and totally focus their attention on an image or images in their mind's eye that they have chosen to concentrate on. There are documented cases in which people have used visualization to reduce or eliminate pain associated with tumors, cancer, and arthritis; to eliminate phobias; and to manage various mental conditions.

Guided imagery is the technique used to take the mental "trip" through your scene. Visualization (I use this term to refer to guided imagery as well throughout this section) can be a very powerful healing technique. You can learn it on your own from self-help books or tapes, or you can study with someone who gives private or group sessions. Many people use visualization as part of their therapy for serious diseases, such as cancer and AIDS, to create images that help them eliminate or reduce their pain and create healing. You can do the same for your back pain.

## Visualization for Your Back Pain

William Fezler, a psychotherapist and author of *Creative Imagery: How to Visualize in All Five Senses,* explains a visualization method of pain control called negative hallucination in which you do not experience something that is really there. Have you ever stared right at something you were looking for—your keys or your glasses, for example—and not seen them? This is an example of a negative visual hallucination. For pain you can create a negative tactile hallucination—you can imagine that the pain or the painful area does not exist.

You may want to tape the following brief visualization. It leads you through deep breathing to prepare you for a popular visualization—a beach scene—but you can use whatever scene you can vividly re-create in your mind. Once you strengthen your imaging abilities—and this may take several sessions—you can go on to create a negative hallucination. Set aside about fifteen to twenty minutes in a place you won't be disturbed. If you tape this example, pause five or more seconds at each ellipsis ( . . . ).

As you breathe in, your mind is becoming clearer and clearer . . . every time you breathe out, your mind becomes lighter. Continue to inhale slowly and deeply, filling your mind with light . . . continue to exhale slowly and gently, releasing any tension with every molecule of breath.

Take a deep breath, and as you let it out, know that there is a light somewhere in your mind . . . Focus on the light and see how it shimmers. Feel the warmth coming from the light . . . in your mind's eye, reach out to the light . . . breathe into the light . . . this is where the mind and the body meet. Welcome the warmth and the light . . . acknowledge that they are a part of you.

Continue to breathe naturally and gently . . . You are now going on a journey to a place you may or may not have been before . . . but you will be there now. You are walking on a beach. The sun has just peeked up over the horizon and is casting a carpet of light on the water.

The sky is ablaze with color—gold, orange, blue, pink—that tinges the puffs of clouds that dot the sky. Feel the warmth of the new sun on your face as you walk along the beach . . . Feel the damp, cool sand between your toes and beneath your bare feet . . . Walk to the water's edge and feel the shock of cold water as the waves sweep up over your feet . . . Hear the waves crash on the shore and the swoosh of water as they leave.

Breathe in the cool salt air . . . focus on how it feels in your nose and in your lungs . . . listen to the songs of the gulls as they fly over the waves and over the sand . . . hear as their calls grow louder and then softer as they swoop near and then away from you . . . the sun is overhead now . . . feel the heat from the sun on your skin. As you look out to the ocean, see how the light dances on the water. Notice how it sparkles and casts diamonds of light on the ocean's surface . . . Stare at the light and breathe into it . . . feel your skin tingle with the energy you take in from the light.

As you continue to breathe and stare at the light, notice that it is beginning to change . . . Now the sun is lower in the sky and there are purple and green dots on the water . . . As the sun sinks lower in the sky, you feel more and more relaxed. When the sun reaches the horizon, see the many colors in the sky—red, gold, scarlet, orange, blue, crimson—and feel a sense of calm. Continue to breathe deeply and gently.

As the sun sets, you feel an incredible sense of peace and relaxation . . . Watch as the sun sinks into the horizon, drawing all of its colors along with it from the sky. You are now enveloped with the cloak of night . . . You are wonderfully relaxed . . .

Once you can create this or a scene of your choice so vividly that you believe you are there, imagine you are in the scene and doing something you are unable to do now because of your pain—swimming or building a sand castle if you are on the beach; or it may be playing tennis, gardening, skiing, or whatever pleasant activity you choose. See yourself moving in this activity as if your pain does not exist. This is your negative hallucination. Imagine the scene so clearly that you can smell the sea air as you swim and feel the sting of the salt on your skin, for example. Stay in your scene for several minutes if you can, moving as if the pain were not there. To bring yourself out, tell yourself, "I am going to count to five. When I reach five, I will open my eyes and be totally relaxed."

Practice the entire visualization sequence three times a day for about ten minutes each time, and you should begin to move with less pain or no pain after about a week, depending on your pain level and your persistence. Soon you should be able to go directly to the negative-hallucination part of your visualization without going through the creation of the beach scene and use it to help control pain at any time during the day. Simply set aside a minute to take a deep breath, focus on the images you have created time and time again, and be in that space of no pain.

Another visualization technique is to imagine the pain leaving you. Robin, an elementary school teacher, uses this approach for acute back pain to help her get through a full day of teaching. She practices visualization before classes, during lunch, and takes two or three five-minute breaks during the day. In her visualization she "surgically" removes the place in her back where the pain is, wraps it up in yards and yards of paper and tape "so it can't get out," weights it with bricks, and tosses it over the Golden Gate Bridge. Other visualizations that have worked for people include packing the pain in a suitcase and sending it on a plane (this by a disgruntled traveler who says the airlines will certainly lose the luggage), and sending the pain up in a spacecraft to hurdle endlessly out into the universe.

## How Does Visualization Work?

Scientists tell us that visual, auditory, and tactile (touch) imagery are produced in the cerebral cortex, the thinking and language center of the brain. Using a technique called *positron emission tomography (PET),* which maps brain activity, researchers have found that the cerebral cortex is equally activated whether people actually experience something or if they just create a vivid image in their mind. In other words the brain "thinks" the images are real, but they're not. The brain registers the picture and sends messages to the other bodily systems, including the autonomic nervous system, which regulates temperature, blood pressure, and heart rate. The body gets the message, and changes occur: Serotonin levels—the body's natural relaxation chemical—increase while heart rate and breathing rate decrease. You enter a state of relaxation, which increases your pain threshold, as compared with anxiety and stress, which reduce your tolerance for pain. The more vividly you imagine a scene, the more effective your session will be.

# YOGA

From its origins in India among the Hindus to the living rooms of Anytown, U.S.A., the practice of yoga has spread around the world. There are several types of yoga, most of which focus on spiritual enlightenment. Hatha yoga, however, combines physical healing with meditation—a mind-body approach. As you stretch, strengthen, and heal your body using gentle movements and biomechanically correct alignment, your mind focuses in a meditative way on your breathing, movements, and physical sensations. Your mind and body work as one to heal. And it seems that many people concur. According to the 1983–84 Yoga Biomedical Trust survey, 98 percent of more than 1,100 people with back pain reported beneficial effects from yoga.

For Alicia, a forty-two-year-old CPA, yoga provides a sense of awareness. "The more I practice yoga, the more I understand what my body is saying to me," she says. "I had chronic back pain for seven years, but several months after I started yoga, the pain was nearly gone. I'm stronger and more flexible now than I was ten years ago. When I get stressed and my muscles tense up, yoga brings me back to a relaxed place. The pain subsides, my mind is quiet, and I can continue to work."

## Yoga and Your Back Pain

Before you begin a yoga program, you need to assess your flexibility and alignment and discuss your plans with your doctor or other health care professional. If you have scoliosis, a herniated disk, or other specific back condition or if you are pregnant, there are some positions you should avoid. Once you know the condition of your back, you can choose which yoga positions you want to try. For some that means accessing books and videos and learning yoga on their own or getting a few private lessons from a yoga instructor who has worked with people with back pain. For others it means joining a class led by a trained yoga instructor. If you choose the former, review the sources in "Suggestions for Further Reading" and Appendix B. After you learn some of the basics, you may want to join a beginner's class.

The three yoga poses explained in this section are for beginners. They are designed to gently stretch tight muscles, strengthen weak ones, and improve posture. Do them slowly and do not push yourself. Practice these and other beginning poses daily for several months before you move ahead to more advanced poses. Read "Yoga Prep and Tips" before you get started.

---

### YOGA PREP AND TIPS

- Wear comfortable clothing that allows you to see what your body is doing. Shorts and a T-shirt, a leotard, or a swimsuit are fine; sweat pants are not.
- Bare feet are the rule—and comfortable, too.
- You will need the following accessories:

  1. Head- and neck-support rolls (folded or rolled-up hand towels for the neck; bath towel for the head).

  2. Lumbar pad (folded bath towel).

  3. Blankets (wool or heavy cotton are best).

  4. A nonskid mat if you are not practicing on a nonskid floor. Proper alignment of your head, neck, and back are important, so experiment with the placement and thickness of the rolls and pads until you are comfortable.

- To derive the most benefit from yoga, you need to practice proper breathing. This means:

  1. Inhale and exhale through your nose.

  2. As you inhale, relax the muscles in your face, neck, and shoulders and focus on maintaining correct posture.

  3. As you exhale, perform the action of the pose.

  4. Never hold your breath.

  5. If you focus on your breathing during your yoga sessions, you bring in the benefits of meditation—stress reduction and increased self-awareness.

- Set aside fifteen to thirty minutes a day, at least five days

---

a week, for yoga. If you only have five minutes to spend one day, five minutes is better than nothing.

## Pose 1: Crocodile Twist

*Props:* Head pad and neck-support roll.

Lie on your back and position your head pad and neck-support roll. Bend your right knee and place your right foot on top of your left knee. Roll over onto your left side until your right knee touches the floor. Place your left hand on your right knee to hold your knee steady (see Figure II-30). Lower your right shoulder toward the floor and away from your right ear. Reach out with your right arm toward the ceiling and then back behind your body. If you can touch the floor, fine; if not, let your arm go as far as is comfortable. While you are doing this, stretch out your left leg through the heel and pull the toes back toward you. Stay in this position for thirty to sixty seconds and breathe normally.

Visualize your spine and imagine that it is lengthening and the muscles are relaxing.

To come out of the pose, lift your right arm up and point it toward the ceiling as you exhale. Slowly roll over onto your back and note how your back feels.

Repeat the pose on the other side and do two to three more complete sets.

This pose gently increases the space between the vertebrae by lengthening the paraspinal muscles. NOTE: Do not attempt this pose during the second half of pregnancy.

## Pose 2: Easy Bridge Pose

*Prop:* One folded blanket.

Lie on your back and place the blanket under your shoulders. Bend your knees and place your feet parallel, flat on the floor, with your heels close to your buttocks and about

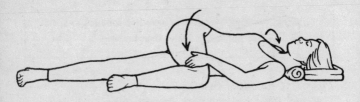

**II-30    Yoga pose: crocodile twist**

hip-width apart. Rest your arms at your sides, palms up. On an exhale, use your abdominal muscles to press your lower back into the floor, tilting your pelvis. Hold this pose as you inhale. On the next exhale, slowly lift your buttocks by pressing your feet firmly into the floor—and maintain the pelvic tilt! Raise your buttocks six to eight inches off the floor as you continue to breathe easily (see note below). Keep your eyes looking toward your knees. To prevent your weight from shifting to the outer edge of your feet, press down with your inner heels. Keep your knees hip-width apart and your shoulders and face relaxed.

Hold this position for several seconds, then return to the starting position on an exhale. Maintain the pelvic tilt as you lower your hips.

Repeat the sequence three to six times (see Figure II-31).

This pose strengthens the abdominals, hamstrings, and buttock muscles, as well as stretches the hip flexors and improves increased lumbar curves. NOTE: If you have spondylolysis or spondylolisthesis, lift your buttocks no more than three inches from the floor. Also do not practice this pose during the second half of pregnancy.

### Pose 3: One Leg Up, One Leg Out

*Props:* Neck-support roll, head pad; lumbar pad and rolled blanket if needed.

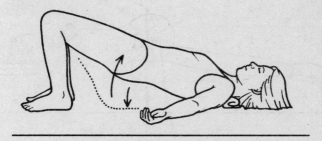

**II-31   Yoga pose: easy bridge pose**

Practice this pose in a doorway or anywhere you can stretch one leg up the wall and the other straight on the floor. Begin by sitting with your left side close to the wall. Place your forearms on the floor as you lie down and extend your left leg up the wall. Position your head and neck supports and place your arms at your sides. Keep your right leg bent with the foot on the floor.

Position your buttocks to allow your left leg to straighten completely and your sacrum to press on the floor (see Figure II-32A). If your left leg is not straight, move your buttocks away from the wall until you can straighten your leg (see Figure II-32B). You should feel a hamstring stretch in your left leg. Hold this pose for two to five minutes.

Repeat the sequence for the other leg. Once the left leg is straight, slowly stretch out your right leg. If this position bothers your lower back, place a rolled blanket behind your knee (Figure II-32B).

This pose stretches the hamstrings and hip flexors and is very good if you have scoliosis, spondylolysis, or spondylolisthesis. NOTE: Use a lumbar pad if you have a flat back. Avoid this pose during the second half of pregnancy.

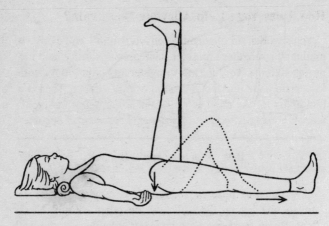

**II-32A    One leg up, one leg out**

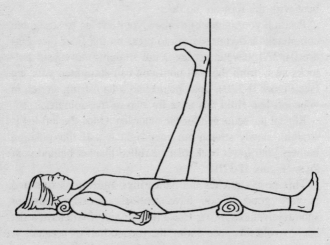

**II-32B    pose for those with limited flexibility**

## How Does Yoga Help Alleviate Back Pain?

Yoga works simultaneously on your mind and body. It gradually strengthens muscles, increases flexibility, and improves stamina. You'll stand straighter and taller, move with less or no pain, and feel a general overall vitality. Yoga is a real boost for the mind as well. When you focus and meditate on your breathing and movements, your mind becomes quiet and tension is relieved. You will experience inner strength and confidence, for when you feel better about yourself, your physical body feels better too.

# PART III

# MEDICAL THERAPIES
# FOR BACK PAIN

Sometimes drugs or other medical interventions will be an appropriate choice for you. In this section we introduce some medical options for back pain: first a description of some common prescription and over-the-counter drugs, their adverse effects, and some precautions to consider; then we briefly describe some of the medical procedures that are used to treat more severe back pain. None of this information is meant to replace that available from your physician or pharmacist. Also please be sure to consult your doctor before self-administering any therapy if you have a specific medical condition.

## THE BACK-PAIN MEDICINE CABINET: DRUGS

Here we open the door to four categories of drugs commonly used for back-pain relief: analgesics, muscle relaxants, antidepressants, and nonsteroidal anti-inflammatory drugs (NSAIDs). AS A GENERAL RULE: If you are currently taking any prescription or nonprescription medication or a homeopathic or herbal remedy, consult your physician or pharmacist before you start a new remedy or drug, even aspirin. Drug interactions can be serious. Also note that any dosages mentioned in the following section are guidelines only. ALWAYS follow package directions or the prescription given to you by your physician or pharmacist.

## Analgesics

Analgesics are typically referred to as painkillers. They are available either in nonnarcotic (acetaminophen) or narcotic (codeine, meperidine, oxycodone) form.

• *Acetaminophen* is taken for mild to moderate pain and is an ingredient in more than one hundred pain formulas; for example, Tylenol, Datril, Panadol, and Anacin-3. Unlike aspirin and other NSAIDs (see page 245), acetaminophen does not reduce inflammation. It is considered to be safer than aspirin and usually does not cause stomach irritation. Most people can take acetaminophen along with an NSAID without experiencing ill effects. Rare cases of kidney or liver damage do occur. If you have liver disease, tell your physician before taking acetaminophen. Less serious adverse effects include diarrhea, rash, loss of appetite, painful urination, and gastrointestinal upset.

• *Narcotic analgesics* are addictive and are usually reserved to treat moderate to severe pain. Narcotic analgesics should not be used to treat chronic low back pain. In addition to their potential for abuse, narcotic analgesics come with a long list of precautions. For example, before taking any narcotic, let your physician know if you have liver, heart, or respiratory disease; if you are pregnant; if you have had a recent head injury; or if you have asthma or epilepsy.

The narcotic analgesics listed below have the potential to

cause drowsiness, constipation, nausea, and dizziness. Additional complications associated with these drugs are given as well.

- **Meperidine** (Demerol). Can cause vomiting, loss of appetite, slow heart rate, difficulty breathing, and fainting.
- **Pentazocine** (Talwin). Associated with hallucinations, confusion, and difficulty breathing.
- **Propoxyphene** (Darvon). Adverse effects include liver damage, confusion, and difficulty breathing.
- **Aspirin + acetaminophen + oxycodone** (Percocet, Vicodin, Percodan). Shortness of breath and slow heart rate can occur.
- **Acetaminophen + codeine** (Tylenol with Codeine). The "with codeine" tag warns you that use of this drug can lead to drug dependence. Side effects include fainting, liver damage, slow heart rate, and difficulty breathing.

## Antidepressants

About thirty years ago researchers discovered that tricyclic antidepressants (the most widely used class of antidepressants) were effective against chronic pain in people with or without depression. The exact reason for this action is still being researched. One theory is that tricyclic antidepressants increase the potency of serotonin, and low serotonin concentrations are associated with chronic pain. When antidepressants are given for pain relief, the doses are significantly lower than those prescribed for depression. A depression dose of imipramine, for example, is 200 mg; for pain, 10 to 75 mg. Some of the newer antidepressants, such as sertraline, bupropion, and fluoxetine, are still being studied for their pain-relief abilities.

Some of the tricyclic antidepressants prescribed for back pain are listed below. All are most effective when taken on an empty stomach but can be taken with a little food if stomach upset is a problem. All have the potential to cause sedation.

- **Amitriptyline** (Elavil). This drug is widely prescribed for chronic back pain. It is the least expensive of the antidepressants and has more side effects than other drugs in this category. People who take amitriptyline for back pain can usually significantly reduce their dose of analgesics. Adverse effects include morning drowsiness, cardiac arrhythmias, blurred vision, dry mouth, weight gain, nausea, rash, and increased perspiration. Individuals who have glaucoma, diabetes, liver disorders, cardiac dysrhythmias, epilepsy, or prostate hypertrophy should avoid using this drug. Imipramine may be a suitable alternative. If sleeping problems exist, amitriptyline is a good choice.
- **Doxepin** (Sinequan, Adapin). This drug is also effective against chronic back pain. Its side effects and precautions are similar to those of amitriptyline. Like amitriptyline, it is useful for people with sleep disturbances.
- **Imipramine** (Tofranil, Trimipramine). Imipramine is generally not as effective as amitriptyline, although it causes some of the same adverse effects. Sudden withdrawal from the drug may cause nausea, malaise, and headache.
- **Nortriptyline** (Pamelor, Aventyl). Adverse effects like those of amitriptyline. Consult your physician before taking any other drug along with nortriptyline, including over-the-counter medications.

## Muscle Relaxants

Muscle relaxants are prescribed to treat spasms, which are involuntary contractions of muscle. Not all physicians believe muscle relaxants should be taken by people with back pain. Some insist spasm is a natural reaction muscle uses to heal itself; others say there is very little evidence that muscle relaxants are effective. Another argument against their use is that many of these drugs do not work on the muscles but on the central nervous system, where they modify muscle tone. Still other physicians point out that many muscle relaxants have serious side effects, including drowsiness, addiction, and insomnia. It's also important to know that muscle relaxants alone do not relieve pain, which means you need to take other steps to deal with the pain.

On a more positive note muscle relaxants can help people who have trouble sleeping because of muscle pain. For individuals with acute back pain, the sedation caused by muscle relaxants helps them rest, although they should be up and active after two days. Medications that combine a muscle relaxant and an analgesic are more effective than a muscle relaxant alone in controlling muscle spasm.

If your doctor prescribes muscle relaxants, ask questions about what you can expect from their use. Below are some common muscle relaxants and comments about each:

- **Carisoprodol** (Carisoprodate, Rela, Sodol, Soma Compound). This drug can cause extreme weakness, loss of balance, loss of vision, agitation, irritability, headache, depression, insomnia, rapid heartbeat, flushing, vomiting, hiccups, increased tissue swelling, rash, drowsiness, dizziness, nausea, and allergic reactions. Soma contains aspirin and is best taken with meals. Headache and insomnia may occur if you suddenly stop taking this drug.

- **Cyclobenzaprine** (Flexeril). Adverse effects include dry mouth, drowsiness, euphoria, depression, headache, nightmares, insomnia, dizziness, numbness, tingling, visual disturbances, and seizures. Do not take if you have glaucoma, prostatic hypertrophy, an overactive thyroid, or myocardial infarction.

- **Chlorzoxazone** (Paraflex, Parafon Forte). Can cause anemia, drowsiness, excitement, loss of appetite, heartburn, upset stomach, dizziness, liver damage, or allergic reactions such as rash or itching. Parafon Forte contains acetaminophen. Chlorzoxazone can cause urine to turn orange or purple.

- **Diazepam** (Valium, Zetran). Prolonged use of diazepam can cause depression, while abrupt cessation of the drug is associated with withdrawal symptoms. Drowsiness is its primary side effect; others include dizziness, clumsiness, extreme weakness, difficulty breathing, slurred speech, tremor, slow heartbeat, disturbed vision, and confusion. Diazepam can be highly addictive.

- **Metaxalone** (Skelaxin). Drowsiness, upset stomach, fast or slow heartbeat, fainting, hives, rash, stinging eyes, and stuffy nose are the minor side effects; liver damage, allergic reactions, and decreased blood cell count may also occur. If your skin turns yellow or you get a rash while on metaxalone, contact your doctor.

- **Methocarbamol** (Delaxin, Marbaxin, Robaxin). Destruction of red blood cells, blurred vision, dizziness, headache, low blood pressure, faintness, seizures, loss of appetite, metallic taste, blood clots, slow heartbeat, and allergic reactions can result from use of this drug. Methocarbamol can also turn your urine black, green, or brown. If a rash, fever, itching, or nasal congestion develop, contact your physician. Do not take if you have impaired kidney function, epilepsy, myasthenia gravis, or are taking anticholinesterase drugs.

- **Orphenadrine** (Banflex, Disipal, Flexagin, Norflex, Norgesic). The Norgesic formulation contains aspirin and caffeine. Orphenadrine can cause anemia, rapid heartbeat, irritability, dry mouth, weakness, blurred vision, urine retention, drowsiness, dizziness, palpitations, fainting, and allergic reactions. It should not be taken if you have glaucoma; enlarged prostate; duodenal, bowel, or bladder-neck obstruction; rapid heartbeat; severe liver or kidney dysfunction; or ulcerative colitis.

## Nonsteroidal Anti-inflammatory Drugs (NSAIDs)

Aspirin is the most well-known and the most economical drug in this category, which consists of more than two dozen agents. The primary function of NSAIDs is to reduce swelling, with analgesia (pain reduction) as a secondary feature. Not all NSAIDs effectively reduce pain. When NSAIDs are used as analgesics, they must usually be taken every four to six hours. Exceptions are diflunisal, piroxicam, and naproxen; consult your physician before taking these drugs.

The most common side effects of NSAIDs are bleeding stomach lining, peptic ulcers, bruising, fluid retention, dizziness, ringing in the ears, and nausea. Each NSAID may also have specific drug interactions and precautions. Before you take any of these drugs, ALWAYS consult with your doctor or pharmacist to learn about contraindications.

- **Aspirin.** Dozens of over-the-counter pain medications contain aspirin. It inhibits the body's production of some prostaglandins, the chemical mediators of inflammation—swelling, redness, heat, and pain—which stimulate the nerve cells that carry the pain signals to the brain. When the body releases the chemical serotonin into the bloodstream, which causes the blood vessels to expand, aspirin moves in to help keep serotonin levels down.

Prostaglandins are responsible for maintaining a healthy stomach lining. Aspirin inhibits prostaglandin production and can irritate your stomach, so take it with food. The enteric form, which provides a coating that does not dissolve until the drug reaches the stomach, can still cause stomach irritation because the aspirin enters the stomach lining via the bloodstream.

- **Ibuprofen** (Advil, Medipren, Midol, Motrin, Nuprin, Rufen). This over-the-counter drug is available in 200-mg strength tablets; higher-dose formulas are available by prescription. Avoid ibuprofen if you cannot tolerate aspirin. Ibuprofen has fewer side effects than aspirin but can cause rash, itching, upset stomach, blurred vision, ulcers, ringing in the ears, decreased appetite, fluid retention, bleeding, and dizziness. Large doses taken over a long period of time may lead to kidney damage. Ibuprofen interacts with many other drugs and increases the risk of bleeding and peptic ulcer. When self-medicating, do not take more than 1.2 g per day.
- **Indomethacin** (Indocin). This NSAID also has analgesic and fever-reducing benefits and is the drug of choice for treatment of spondylitis. Of all the NSAIDs this one is the most likely to cause central nervous system toxicity. Potential adverse side effects include anemia, headache, dizziness, depression, drowsiness, confusion, peripheral nerve damage, seizures, faintness, high blood pressure, edema, blurred vision, eye damage, hearing loss, nausea, vomiting, loss of appetite, diarrhea, severe gastrointestinal bleeding, bloody

urine, rash, hives, kidney dysfunction, and peptic ulcers. Great caution should be used if given to anyone with ulcers, bleeding problems, or an allergy to aspirin. Indomethacin may aggravate Parkinson's disease, emotional problems, or epilepsy. Weight gain may occur, as indomethacin causes sodium retention.

- **Ketorolac** (Toradol). This nonaddictive NSAID is used for short-term pain management—no longer than five days. The typical dose is 30 mg. It comes in an injectable (side effects include ulcerations, bleeding, and perforation of the gastrointestinal tract) and an oral form (heartburn, nausea, gastrointestinal pain, and headache). Do not take ketorolac if you are allergic to aspirin, if you have nasal polyps, or you are nursing. Consult your physician before taking ketorolac if you have heart disease, high blood pressure, a history of alcohol abuse, kidney problems, or are taking anticoagulants.
- **Meclofenamate** (Meclomen). This drug has some pain- and fever-relief action. Daily dosage should not exceed 400 mg. Up to 33 percent of patients get diarrhea from this drug. Other side effects include anemia, fatigue, insomnia, water retention, dizziness, nervousness, headache, blurred vision, abdominal pain, hives, nausea, hemorrhage, painful and/or bloody urine, and kidney or liver toxicity. Avoid use if you have ulcers, asthma, diabetes, blood problems, or liver, kidney, or heart disease.
- **Naproxen sodium** (Anaprox, Naprosyn). Like meclofenamate, this drug also has analgesic and fever-reducing effects. Naproxen sodium usually acts within twenty minutes of ingestion, and the sodium form is absorbed more readily than naproxen alone. Abdominal pain, peptic ulcer, nausea, and gas are the most common side effects. Others include low white blood

count, dizziness, drowsiness, shortness of breath, headache, water retention, rash, hemorrhage, hives, kidney toxicity, and liver toxicity. Do not take naproxen sodium if you have asthma and nasal polyps. Caution is emphasized if you are elderly, are allergic to NSAIDs, have gastrointestinal disorders, or have heart or kidney disease.

- **Phenylbutazone** (Butazolidin). Take this drug exactly as prescribed, as it can cause serious side effects, especially in people older than forty. Maximum dosage is 400 mg.

## INJECTION THERAPY

When other pain-management measures fail, some people turn to injection therapy. This method involves injecting an anesthetic, corticosteroid, or other substance into a disk, joint, or soft tissue. Studies have been done of various injection therapies. Many results support its use, while many others show conflicting findings. Since these dissenting reports are usually based on studies that were poorly designed, their findings cannot be used either to prove or to disprove the therapy's effectiveness. Therefore injection therapies as a whole are controversial.

### Analgesics—Local Injections

Local injections of analgesics into painful muscles or ligaments are frequently made by physicians for patients with low back pain. These injections are for pain caused by inflamed muscles or joints or for a fibromyositis. The injected substances may include plain saline, local anesthetics alone, or local anesthetics combined with a cortisone (see Glossary) preparation. Such injections typically mask the pain for a short time, if at all, and do not address the cause of the pain.

## Chymopapain

Chymopapain is an enzyme extracted from papaya that is injected into the spine to treat herniated disks. Once chymopapain enters the disk, it dissolves the nucleus and relieves the pressure exerted by the disk against a nerve. This procedure is called chemonucleosis. The basic procedure goes like this: Before you receive a chymopapain treatment, you will get a general anesthetic, followed by the injection. About 50 percent of people experience severe temporary back pain after the injection. Some people go home after they wake up from the anesthesia; others stay in the hospital for a few days.

Chymopapain injection is controversial. Physicians who support it say it is successful in 75 percent of patients, whereas surgery is effective in only 60 percent. They also point out that it is simpler than surgery and less expensive. Opponents of chymopapain admit that 75 percent of patients who receive the injections have less pain after the procedure, but they argue that surgery has a much higher success rate.

Not everyone is a candidate for this treatment. If you have asthma, have ever experienced severe allergic reactions, are allergic to papaya or meat tenderizers, have had a chymopapain injection previously, or have other spinal cord problems, it's not for you. About 1 percent of people do have a severe allergic reaction to the injection. Other potential side effects include paralysis, stroke, nausea, headache, weakness or numbness in the legs, stiffness, back spasm, and dizziness.

## DMSO

Dimethyl sulfoxide—DMSO—is a by-product of paper-making and is available in commercial and pharmaceutical grades. The pharmaceutical formula is used by osteopaths and naturopaths in intravenous injections to treat sciatica and lumbar disk problems, as well as other medical problems. A 20 percent solution of DMSO is combined with the local anesthetic Xylocaine and injected into painful back areas, including diseased spinal disks, to eliminate pain.

To get lasting relief, DMSO needs to be injected on three to five consecutive days. DMSO can also be applied full strength on the skin over an area of pulled muscles for pain relief, although it can cause a burning sensation. Another side effect of DMSO is its odor, which is similar to rotten garlic.

## Epidural Cortisone

This treatment is used in patients who have not responded to other therapies for herniated disk, spinal stenosis, lumbar nerve root compression, and other inflammatory conditions. Injection of cortisone plus a small amount of a local anesthetic into the epidural (*epi* means "outside"; *dura* is the lining membrane of the spinal cord) has an antiinflammatory effect on the nerve root and the surrounding tissue. Epidural injections are also effective in some cases of sciatica. Overall a 40 percent successful-response rate is associated with this therapy, and relief is usually only temporary.

Epidural corticosteroid injection is considered safe if the physician is extremely careful with his technique. Potential complications include various types of meningitis and arachnoiditis (inflammation of the arachnoid membrane).

## Facet Joint

People who have arthritis that is causing chronic back pain that has not responded to other conservative treatment may opt for facet-joint injection. A complete treatment usually requires that three injections of cortisone and a local anesthetic be made every two to four weeks. Injections are made into the joints both above and below the affected joint in order to get adequate pain relief. Facet-joint injection is a controversial therapy, and no studies have shown that it provides long-term pain relief.

## Peripheral Nerve Block

People with chronic pain who have not gotten relief from other courses of therapy, including oral medications, may consider peripheral nerve block. Specific nerves, such as the sciatic nerve, as well as selected areas, may be treated. If you elect this type of therapy, you will receive a series of three injections, usually on an outpatient basis. As soon as you feel improvement, which can be within twelve to twenty-four hours of the injection, increase your physical activity.

## Sclerosant

A combination of carefully placed sclerosant injections and a postinjection exercise program is successful in some patients with chronic low back pain. The injection, composed of dextrose, glycerine, and phenol, helps strengthen connective tissues by promoting the formation of collagen, a protein found in such tissue. Sclerosant injections should be given by a physician who has much experience with this procedure.

# SURGERY

Say "back surgery" and most people shudder. Perhaps they should, especially if they consider that many of the approximately quarter-million back surgeries done every year to remove herniated disks and tens of thousands of other back operations performed for other conditions could have been avoided.

Many physicians believe surgery should be a last resort, after all other feasible alternatives and methods have been tried. According to Dr. Hochschuler of the Texas Back Institute, surgery should be considered only after the following approaches have been pursued: physical examination, physical therapy, hydrotherapy, extensive exercise, back school, biofeedback, injections, and diagnostic tests to determine the need for surgery. If you believe your doctor has prescribed back surgery without considering enough alternatives, we recommend you get a second opinion.

Surgery is not a silver bullet; even after a herniated disk is removed or spinal fusion has been done, a daily movement program needs to be followed if recurrence of back pain is to be avoided. Many people who undergo back surgery faithfully do their physical therapy for a while and then incorrectly believe they are "cured."

Here are some of the common back-surgery procedures.

## Diskectomy

In people with a severe herniated disk, an open (conventional) diskectomy can be done to remove part of the disk that is affecting the nearby nerves. The remainder of the disk is left intact so that it can continue to function. This procedure yields good to excellent results (90 to 95 percent success rate) initially, but recurrence or scarring brings this rate down to 70 percent within a decade of the procedure.

## Microdiskectomy

This procedure involves the use of a 2.5 to 3.0 cm incision and a high-powered microscope. It is more economical than open diskectomy because of its shorter hospital stay, although recovery time is similar. This procedure relieves leg pain in about 90 percent of cases, and back pain in fewer. Although this procedure allows patients to return to daily activities faster, many surgeons are not convinced microdiskectomy is better than the conventional operation because it does not permit them to adequately view the area for disk fragments, which may lead to the need for reoperation.

## Percutaneous Diskectomy

A newer type of procedure is percutaneous diskectomy, which can be done under local anesthesia. The disk fragments are "sucked" out through a narrow tube inserted through a tiny incision and into the damaged area. A local anesthetic is all that is required, and the incision is covered with a bandage. The procedure does not require an overnight stay, and most patients are active within one week. One concern about this procedure is making sure all fragments are removed, as those left behind can cause problems later. This and similar procedures are currently under investigation.

## Fusion

In some cases of degenerative disk disease or badly worn facet joints, a surgeon may fuse two or more vertebrae together. To do this, bone from the patient's pelvis or from a bone bank is grafted to the vertebrae. As the graft heals, a bridge develops and stabilizes the area. It may take up to a year for the bridge to form, and a brace is usually needed to help reduce postoperative pain, which can be great, and to reinforce the area. Although the word *fusion* leads many people to believe the operation will leave them with an unbendable spine, patients usually do not notice any loss of function or movement in the back. Researchers are still uncertain about the exact indications for spinal fusion; therefore it is used only in carefully selected cases.

## Foramenotomy

Individuals with spinal stenosis (narrowing of the spinal canal) may get relief from this procedure. Small openings in the vertebrae, called foramen, allow the spinal nerves to pass through. When these passageways become inflamed or swollen, a surgeon may need to shave the bone around the foramen. This opens up the space and reduces inflammation.

## Rhizotomy

For individuals with facet-joint pain, the surgeon cuts the nerves of the vertebral facet joint, thereby interrupting the pain signal to the brain.

## Scoliosis Correction

The best time to correct scoliosis is during childhood and adolescence, when the spine is more flexible. Mild cases can be treated with movement therapy; moderate curves usually require that the child wear a brace. If the curvature is severe, or if the problem was not addressed until adulthood, surgical spine straightening can be done. Instruments called Cotrel-Dubousset rods, introduced in the United States in 1985, untwist and straighten the spine in a corkscrewlike fashion. Harrington rods, in use since 1962, stretch out the curvature in the spine. Surgeons are reluctant to perform these procedures on adults because the spine is more brittle and less flexible with age.

# TENS

A transcutaneous electrical nerve stimulation (TENS) device is a small power unit that delivers minute amounts of electrical current to a body site that is painful. It is a safe therapy for both acute and chronic pain, and it is especially useful for people who have gotten little or no relief from medications. TENS is frequently used by people who are recovering from back surgery, and it also offers relief to individuals with sciatica.

The TENS device is simple to use: Clip the beeper-sized unit to your belt and run the wire leads with electrodes at the ends under your clothing to the treatment sites (see Figure III-1). Your physician will place the electrodes based on the location and type of your pain. Don't be surprised if it takes several "test runs" before the most effective locations are found, because it isn't possible to predict the optimal sites. The electrodes are usually placed on or around the area of maximum pain or near the nerves that go into the painful area. Trigger points associated with muscle pain are often the same as acupuncture points. The closer the electrodes are to the nerve, the lower the current needed to stimulate the nerve fibers.

Once the unit is turned on—you decide when you need it—a low level of electricity stimulates the nerve fibers and blocks the pain signals to the brain. Some people don't feel this current at all; others report a slight tingling sensation. Individuals with sensitive skin may experience some mild irritation from the electrodes. A word of caution to those

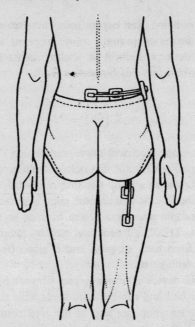

**III-1  A TENS unit positioned for low back pain**

with pacemakers: Check with your physician before using a TENS unit, as the frequencies it emits may disrupt pacemaker function.

## TENS for Your Back Pain

A physician must prescribe TENS for you, but a physical therapist, nurse, or other knowledgeable professional can explain how it works and monitor your progress. Once you are "hooked up," you may experience pain relief almost immediately, or it may take several hours. The average time is twenty minutes. If you have chronic pain, it may take thirty minutes or longer for the benefits to become apparent. This relief may last beyond the actual treatment or only while the unit is operating.

How effective is TENS? During the early stages of therapy, 60 to 80 percent of chronic pain can be reduced. After one year of use, between 20 and 30 percent of users continue to get relief from the stimulation. TENS appears to be as effective as acupuncture and more effective than conventional massage. It also has a placebo effect; about 30 percent of people given sham treatments report having pain relief. However, TENS also produces relief in more than 30 percent of people who have intractable back pain.

TENS works best when you make it a part of your therapy. Natural therapies such as biofeedback and other relaxation techniques, as well as movement therapy and increased awareness of your posture and daily activities (see Chapter 3) can make TENS a good choice for you, especially if you have chronic pain.

## How Does TENS Work?

Experts have several ideas about how TENS works. Some believe it acts as an "off" switch for the transmission of pain messages to the brain; others say the electrical stimulation helps trigger the release of endorphins and enkephalins—the body's natural pain relievers. They do agree, however, that TENS can relieve pain, although it cannot prevent it.

# Summary

Discoveries are being made every day in conventional medicine: new drugs, new uses for existing drugs, improved surgical techniques, advanced diagnostic procedures. At the same time people like yourself are discovering the virtues of natural therapies, many of which are centuries old.

In this book we have shown you that when it comes to your health, especially your back pain, you have three options—not one: conventional medicine, natural medicine, or a combination of the two. Regardless of the path you choose, we strongly recommend you first get a medical examination to rule out any serious condition. Also keep in mind that there is no good correlation between test results and the presence of back pain. Many people with back problems have negative test results, and just as many have positive results. If at any time during your treatment of back pain you experience a worsening of pain or any of the symptoms noted in Chapter 2 under "Do I Need a Doctor?" see your physician immediately.

When you take a natural approach to treating back pain, you establish a dialogue with your body. Christine, a thirty-six-year-old former chronic-back-pain sufferer, calls it an honest approach: "When I was dumping chemicals [drugs] into my body for my pain, I was lying to myself. I didn't know how to deal with the pain, so I covered it up. But it was always there, underneath the drugs. Now I do biofeedback, acupressure, and meditation. When I do have pain, which isn't very often, I approach it head-on and honestly. I'm in control, and that feels good."

And that is our wish for you: Feel good. We hope this book has helped you.

# GLOSSARY

**Acupressure**

Treatment that combines the Japanese method of finger pressure and the Chinese system of acupuncture points and meridians to release muscle tension, relieve pain, and increase circulation.

**Acupuncture**

Treatment that involves the insertion of fine needles along the meridian points to release blocked energy.

**Acute condition**

Characterized by rapid onset; a disorder in which symptoms develop suddenly and then either resolve quickly or need to be treated immediately. Symptoms may be severe.

**Adrenal glands**

An organ, located on top of each kidney, that produces adrenaline and norepinephrine, two substances that regulate blood pressure and heart rate.

**Analgesic**

Any agent that has a pain-relieving action.

**Ankylosing spondylitis**

A type of arthritis in which the vertebrae gradually fuse together until the spine is rigid. Also known as ankylosing spondyloarthrosis, stiff spine, frozen spine, poker spine.

Annulus fibrosus — Latin for "fibrous ring," it is the outer section of an intervertebral disk.

Anti-inflammatory — Any substance that reduces inflammation.

Antispasmodic — Any substance that prevents spasm.

Arthritis — A general term for inflammation of a joint. There are more than one hundred types of arthritis.

Autoimmune — Refers to conditions in which the body produces antibodies against itself.

Backbone — Another name for the spinal column.

Biofeedback — A system that allows people to hear or see how their body responds physically so that they can learn how to consciously produce more positive or beneficial physical changes.

Blockage — The accumulation of energy in or around an acupuncture point. You may feel this blockage as stiffness, pain, numbness, or an ache. An energy blockage can occur when either the vital force or the emotions and feelings are obstructed.

Cartilage — A type of body tissue that is both flexible and somewhat stiff. Cartilage forms the nose and ears as well as the disks in the spine.

CAT scan — Computerized axial tomography. This test uses a scanner to produce three-dimensional X rays that allow physicians to view soft-tissue areas.

| | |
|---|---|
| Central nervous system | The brain and the spinal cord. |
| Cerebrospinal fluid | A clear fluid produced by the brain that bathes the area between the meninges and that serves as a shock absorber for the central nervous system. |
| Cervical spine | The neck region. |
| Chiropractic | A science based on the theory that health and disease are intimately associated with the nervous system and that a misaligned spine can cause problems throughout the body. Chiropractic healing occurs through manipulation of the spine. |
| Chronic condition | Any disorder that is long-lasting and persistent or recurrent; in medicine any condition that lasts longer than three to six months. |
| Coccyx | The bones that make up the tailbone. |
| Compress | A piece of material in a pad form that is soaked in a hot or cold solution and applied to an external body part. |
| Cranial | Relating to the skull, specifically the bones that encase the brain. |
| Disk | A structure composed of a fibrous outer ring and a soft center and that is found between the vertebral bodies. |
| Diskectomy | A surgical procedure that removes an entire disk or its nucleus. |
| Electromyography | EMG; a test in which muscle disorders are diagnosed using needle electrodes that transmit electrical impulses from the muscle tissue into which they are inserted. |

Endorphin

A painkilling substance produced naturally by the body.

Erector spinae

The back muscles that extend the trunk.

Essential oil

The pure, concentrated essence that is extracted from plants.

Extensor muscles

Four muscles that originate on the vertebrae and extend vertically along the spine to stabilize it. These muscles straighten the limbs of the body.

Facet joint

A joint surrounded by synovial fluid, which is formed by the bony protrusions of two adjacent vertebrae.

Fibrositis

A condition in which musculoskeletal tissues are tender; also called fibromyalgia and fibromyositis.

Flexion

The motion of bending a body part.

Gate-control theory

The concept that sensory stimulation blocks pain signals at the spinal cord.

Hamstrings

The muscles located in the back of the thigh; these muscles flex the knee and extend the hip.

Herniated disk

A condition in which part of the nucleus of a disk protrudes through the outer disk wall into the spinal canal. Often referred to as a slipped disk.

Holistic

A concept based on the perspective that everything is connected; that the entire being or entity is greater than the sum of all its parts; and that any one or more parts of a whole has an influence on the whole.

| | |
|---|---|
| Intervertebral | Referring to the area between the vertebrae. |
| Joint | Where the ends of two bones meet and are joined. |
| Lamina | The posterior part of the vertebral arch. |
| Laminectomy | A surgical procedure that involves removal of the lamina; the purpose is to relieve nerve-root compression from a ruptured disk. |
| Lordosis | Also called swayback; concave curve of the spine that usually occurs in the cervical and lumbar areas. |
| Lumbago | Common term for backache. |
| Lumbar | Referring to the lower back area; the lumbar vertebrae are the last five spinal bones above the sacrum. |
| Lumbosacral area | The spot on the lower back where the lumbar vertebrae meet the sacrum. |
| Macrobiotic | A dietary philosophy that emphasizes balancing the yin and yang properties of foods (see Yin and yang). Fifty percent of the diet consists of whole grains; 25 percent, vegetables. Avoided foods include red meat, sugar, dairy, eggs, and coffee. |
| Magnetic resonance imaging | A noninvasive test that uses magnetic waves to make images of soft tissues. |
| Manipulation | A technique in which practitioners adjust the spine, joints, and other tissues; used in chiropractic therapy and osteopathy. |

| | |
|---|---|
| Meditation | A technique by which you focus your attention inward to help develop spiritual, physical, and mental calm and peace. |
| Meninges | The three membranes that surround the spinal cord and the brain. |
| Meridians | Twelve channels that, according to Eastern concepts, are passageways for the body's vital energy. |
| Muscle | A structure composed of elastic fibers that contract when stimulated and that affect the movement of joints, organs, and other body structures. |
| Naturopath | Health care provider who is concerned with nutritional, psychological, and structural aspects of health, and views all as equally important. |
| Neuralgia | A severe pain that is caused by inflamed nerve fibers. |
| Neurological exam | An examination that includes tests to determine nerve function. |
| Neuromuscular massage | A type of osteopathic massage that affects the muscles and the nerves. |
| Osteopath | A physician whose initial training is the same as that of conventional doctors but also includes manipulation. The practice is based on the understanding that the body is an integrated whole and as such needs to be treated as a functioning whole. |
| Palpation | Use of the hands during a physical examination in order to feel for any abnormalities. |

| | |
|---|---|
| Potency/ Potentization | In homeopathy, the dilution of a remedy that increases its power and determines its therapeutic value. |
| Pressure points | Areas on the human body that have a high level of electrical conductivity. |
| Prolapsed disk | Also called a "slipped" disk; a situation in which the intervertebral disk bulges out and can press on a nerve and cause pain. |
| Referred pain | Pain that originates in one location of the body but manifests as pain somewhere else. |
| Sacral | Referring to the sacrum. |
| Sacroiliac joints | Two places on the lower back where the sacrum joins the hipbones. |
| Sacrum | The flat, triangular bone located at the base of the spine. |
| Scoliosis | A sideways curvature of the spine that is apparent when viewed from behind. |
| Shiatsu | A Japanese method of acupressure. |
| Slipped disk | Medically known as a herniated disk or a protruding intervertebral disk. |
| Spinal column | Also called the backbone, this structure is composed of vertebrae and protects the spinal cord. |
| Spinal cord | A collection of nerves that form a cord that runs through the spinal column and into the brain. |
| Subluxation | In the spine, a partial dislocation of the vertebrae. |
| Sutures | In the head, the connective tissue that holds the bones together. |

| | |
|---|---|
| Tai chi chuan | A Chinese movement-based meditative exercise that promotes and maintains harmony of the body and mind. |
| Toxicity | A poisonous reaction that occurs when people ingest an amount of a substance that is greater than they can tolerate safely. |
| Vertebrae | The series of bones that make up the spinal column. |
| Visualization | A creative process during which you form images and focus your thoughts in a positive direction for the purpose of improving one or more aspects of your life. |
| Vital energy | The life force that is present in all things. The three primary forms include (a) the energy that flows through the body's meridians; (b) the energy generated from positive human qualities such as love, devotion, willpower, and positive thinking; and (c) the energy inherent in natural forms, such as wind, rain, gravity, sun, heat, and electricity. Also known as pana, chi, or ki. |
| Yin and yang | According to the Chinese, these are the two opposing forces in the universe; and because we are part of the universe, we also possess yin and yang. Health depends on the balance of yin and yang, which is manifest in the flow of the vital energy (see above), or chi. |

# APPENDIX A

# Organizations to Contact for Further Information

The following organizations and other entities can be contacted for general information, referrals, and educational opportunities. When writing for information, please send a business-size self-addressed stamped envelope.

## General Information

American Association of Naturopathic Physicians
PO Box 2579; Kirkland, WA 98083-2579
(206) 827-6035

American Chronic Pain Association
PO Box 850; Rocklin, CA 95677
(916) 632-0922
Provides information and services (newsletter, workbooks).

American Holistic Health Association
PO Box 17400; Anaheim, CA 92817
(714) 779-6152

American Holistic Medical Association
433 Front Street; Catasauqua, PA 18032
(610) 433-2448

The American Institute of Stress
124 Park Avenue; Yonkers, NY 10703
(800) 24-RELAX
Information about mind-body relationships and the role of stress
in health. Publishes a monthly newsletter available to the public.

Complementary Medicine Networking and Referral Service
4649 Malvern; Tucson, AZ 85711
(602) 323-6291
Answer questions and refer individuals to doctors practicing general and holistic and/or natural medicine.

Office of Alternative Medicine/National Institutes of Health
9000 Rockville Pike; Bethesda, MD 20892
(800) 377-4865

## Acupressure and Acupuncture

American Oriental Bodywork Association
6801 Jericho Turnpike; Syosset, NY 11791
(516) 364-5533
"Hands-on Health Care" catalog and information.

American Association of Acupuncture and Oriental Medicine
433 Front Street; Catasauqua, PA 18032
(610) 433-2448
Send SASE for general information and information on practitioners.

American Academy of Medical Acupuncturists
5820 Wilshire Boulevard, Suite 500; Los Angeles, CA 90036
(213) 937-5514

## Alexander Technique

American Center for the Alexander Technique
129 W. 67th Street; New York, NY 10023
(212) 799-0468

Alexander Technique
North American Society of Teachers of the Alexander Technique
Box 517; Urbana, IL 61801
(800) 473-0629

## Biofeedback

Biofeedback Certification Institute of America
10200 W. 44th Avenue, Suite 304; Wheatridge, CO 80033
(303) 420-2902
Please send SASE for information and names of practitioners.

Life Sciences Institute of Mind/Body Health
2955 S.W. Wanamaker Drive, Suite B; Topeka, KS 66614
(913) 274-8686
Provides outpatient program and general information.

## Chiropractic

Association for Network Chiropractic Spinal Analysis
PO Box 7682; Longmont, CO 80501
(303) 678-8086
Offers referrals, workshops, seminars, journals, newsletters, etc.

The American Chiropractic Association (ACA)
1701 Clarendon Boulevard; Arlington, VA 22209
(703) 276-8800

International Chiropractors Association
1110 N. Glebe Road, Suite 1000; Arlington, VA 22201
(703) 528-5000

## Craniosacral Therapy

Colorado Cranial Institute
466 Marine Street; Boulder, CO 80302
(303) 447-2760

American Academy of Osteopathy
PO Box 750; Newark, OH 43055
(614) 349-8701

The Cranial Academy
3500 Depaw Boulevard; Indianapolis, IN 46268
(317) 879-0713

## Diet/Nutrition

George Ohsawa Macrobiotic Foundation
1511 Robinson Street; Oroville, CA 95965
(916) 533-7703

North American Vegetarian Society
PO Box 72; Dodgerville, NY 13329
(518) 568-7970

Linus Pauling Institute of Science and Medicine
440 Page Mill Road; Palo Alto, CA 94306
(415) 327-4064 (for vitamin-therapy information)

Physicians Committee for Responsible Medicine
PO Box 6322; Washington, DC 20015.
(202) 686-2210

Macrobiotic Center
61 East 86 Street; New York, NY 10028
(212) 505-1010

# Feldenkrais Method

Feldenkrais Guild
Box 489; Albany, OR 97321
(800) 775-2118

The Feldenkrais Foundation
PO Box 70157; Washington, DC 20088
(301) 656-1548

# Hellerwork

Hellerwork, Inc.
406 Berry Street; Mount Shasta, CA 96067
(800) 392-3900

# Herbal Medicine

American Botanical Council
PO Box 201660; Austin, TX 78720
(800) 373-7105

Herb Society of America
9019 Kirtland Chardon Road; Kirtland, OH 44094
(216) 256-0514

# Homeopathy

American Association of Homeopathic Pharmacists
PO Box 11280; Albuquerque, NM 87192

National Center for Homeopathy
801 N. Fairfax, Suite 306; Alexandria, VA 22314
(703) 548-7790

Homeopathic Educational Services
2124 Kittredge Street; Berkeley, CA 94704
(510) 649-0294

International Foundation for Homeopathy
2366 Eastlake Avenue E. #301; Seattle, WA 98102
(206) 324-8230
General information and how to find practitioners in your area.

Homeopathic Academy of Naturopathic Physicians
14653 Graves Road; Mulino, OR 97042
(503) 795-0579

# Hypnosis

Society for Clinical and Experimental Hypnosis
2200 E. Devon Avenue, Suite 291; Des Plaines, IL 60018
(708) 297-3317
Please send SASE for information.

# Massage

American Massage Therapy Association
1130 W. North Shore Avenue; Chicago, IL 60626
(312) 761-AMTA

# Myotherapy

Bonnie Prudden Pain Erasure
3661 N. Campbell, Suite 102; Tucson, AZ 85719
(800) 221-4643

# Osteopathy

American Osteopathic Association
142 E. Ontario Street; Chicago, IL 60611
(312) 280-5800
Provides information and names of practitioners in your area.

# Polarity Therapy

American Polarity Therapy Association
2888 Bluff Street, Suite 149; Boulder, CO 80301
(303) 545-2080

# Reflexology

International Institute of Reflexology
PO Box 12642; St. Petersburg, FL 33733-2642
(813) 343-4811
Information, seminars, training, books, and worldwide referrals.

# Tai Chi

Complementary Medicine Networking and Referral Service
4649 Malvern; Tucson, AZ 85711
(520) 323-6291

# Therapeutic Touch

American Holistic Nurses Association
4101 Lake Boone Trail, Suite 201; Raleigh, NC 27607
(919) 787-5181

# Trager Therapy

Trager Institute
33 Millwood; Mill Valley, CA 4941
(415) 388-2688

# Visualization

Center for Spiritual Awareness
PO Box 7; Lake Rabun Road; Lakemont, GA 30552
(706) 782-4723

Psycho-Acoustic Technology
4536 Genoa Circle; Virginia Beach, VA 23462
(804) 456-9487

The Institute of Transpersonal Psychology
744 San Antonio Road; Palo Alto, CA 94303
(415) 493-4430
Imagery training; external program on certification in mind-body consciousness and wellness workshops.

The Academy for Guided Imagery
PO Box 2070; Mill Valley, CA 94942
(800) 726-2070

# Yoga

International Association of Yoga Therapists
109 Hillside Avenue; Mill Valley, CA 94941
(415) 383-4587
A nonprofit organization that focuses on research and education.

# Newsletters and Supplies

## Diet and Nutrition

*The Nutrition Action Health Letter*
Center for Science in the Public Interest
1875 Connecticut Avenue NW, Suite 300
Washington, DC 20009-5728
(202) 332-9111
Monthly newsletter for the general public.

*Vegetarian Journal*
Vegetarian Resource Group
PO Box 1463; Baltimore, MD 21203
(410) 366-8343
Information about health, nutrition, and the environment.

*Vegetarian Voice*
North American Vegetarian Society
PO Box 72; Dolgeville, NY 13329
(518) 568-7970
Focus: health, compassionate living, and environment; recipes.

*Vegetarian Times*
PO Box 570; Oak Park, IL 60303
(708) 848-8100
Monthly publication; articles on health, nutrition, and cooking.

## Feldenkrais Technique

*Feldenkrais Resources*
(800) 765-1907
Offers home programs on audiotape. Authorized publisher of the work of Dr. Feldenkrais.

*Relaxercise*
(800) 735-7950
Offers audiotapes based on the work of Dr. Feldenkrais.

## Herbs

East Earth Herb, Inc
PO Box 802; Eugene, OR 97402
(800) 827-HERB

The Herb Closet
104 Main Street; Montpelier, VT 05602
(802) 223-0888

Jean's Greens
RR 1, Box 55J; Rensselaerville, NY 12147
(518) 239-8327

Mountain Rose Herbs
PO Box 2000; Redway, CA 95560
(707) 923-7867

Nature's Way
10 Mountain Springs Parkway; Springville, UT 84663
Available in stores.

OSO Herbals
PO Box 50306-278; Tucson, AZ 85703
(520) 624-9225


Terra Firma Botanicals
28653 Sutherlin Lane; Eugene, OR 97405
Fresh and dried herbal extracts; massage oils; $1 catalog.


## Homeopathy

Boericke & Tafel, Inc.
Santa Rosa, CA 95407
Available in stores.


Homeopathic Overnight
4111 Simon Road; Youngstown, OH 44512
(800) ARNICA30
Mail-order homeopathic remedies.


Homeopathic Educational Services
2124 Kittredge Street; Berkeley, CA 94704
(510) 649-0294, information; (800) 359-9051, orders only
Comprehensive catalog of remedies, books, tapes, and cassettes.


Hadas Natural Products, Ltd.
PO Box 48059; Atlanta, GA 30362
(800) 99-HADAS for information and mail orders. Extensive
line of homeopathic remedies. Also look for them in your pharmacy.


## Massage

The Massage Store, Ltd.
PO Box 2247; Boulder, Co 80306
(800) 728-2426 for a Massage Roller

Royal Pyramid, Inc.
414 Manhattan Avenue; Hawthorne, NY 10532
(800) 325-7423
Ask for their catalog of massage supplies and accessories.

*Massage Magazine*
PO Box 1500; Davis, CA 95617
(916) 757-6033
Published bimonthly; massage, bodywork, and related healing
arts.

## Meditation/Visualization Tapes

QuantumQuests
Box 986; Oakview, CA 93022
(800) 772-0090

*Health Journeys,* available on Time Warner Audiobooks
Tapes by Belleruth Naparstek, Image Paths, Inc.
2635 Payne Avenue; Cleveland, OH 44114
(800) 800-8661

The Source Cassette Learning System
Emmet Miller, M.D.
945 Evelyn Street; Menlo Park, CA 94025
(415) 328-7171
Tapes for relaxation, pain relief. Free catalog.

MindBody Health Sciences
22 Lawson Terrace; Scituate, MA 02066
(617) 545-7122
Offers books and tapes for mental health applications.

Mind/Body Health Sciences, Inc.
393 Dixon Road; Boulder, CO 80302-7177
(303) 440-8460
Relaxation cassettes and videos by the Joan and Miroslav
Borysenko.

## Movement Therapy Supplies (Water)

Sprint Rothhammer
Box 5579; Santa Maria, CA 93456
(800) 235-2156
Swimming: dumbbells, kickboards, hand paddles, floats, etc.

Hydro-Fit, Inc.
405 Lincoln Street; Eugene, OR 97401-2516
(800) 346-7295

## Yoga

Himalayan Institute of Yoga, Science and Philosophy
RR1 Box 400; Honesdale, PA 18431
(717) 253-5551
Catalog; also publishes the magazine *Yoga International.*

Samata Yoga and Health Institute
4150 Tivoli Avenue; Los Angeles, CA 90066
(310) 306-8845
Manuals, videos, and audiocassettes; also offers classes.

*Total Yoga* (video)
White Lotus Foundation; Santa Barbara, CA
(805) 964-1944

Tools for Yoga
(201) 966-5311
Call for catalog.

Yoga Props
(415) 285-9642
Call for catalog.

# SUGGESTIONS FOR FURTHER READING

Abraham, Edward, M.D. *Freedom from Back Pain: An Orthopedist's Self-Help Guide.* Emmaus, PA: Rodale, 1986.

*Alternative Medicine: Expanding Medical Horizons. A Report to the National Institutes of Health on Alternative Medical Systems and Practices in the United States.* Washington, DC: U.S. Government Printing Office, 1994.

Altman, Nathaniel. *Everybody's Guide to Chiropractic Health Care.* Los Angeles: J. P. Tarcher, 1990.

American Medical Association. *The AMA Straight-Talk, No-Nonsense Guide to Back Care.* Revised. Mt. Vernon, NY: Consumers Union, 1984.

Anderson, Dale L., M.D. *90 Seconds to Muscle Pain Relief.* Minneapolis, MN: CompCare Publishers, 1992.

Balch, James F., and Phyllis Balch. *Prescription for Nutritional Healing.* Garden City Park, NY: Avery Publishing Group, 1993.

Balogun, J. A., et al. Spinal mobility and muscular strength: Effects of supine- prone-lying back extension exercise training. *Arch. Phys. Rehabil.* 73 (1992): 745.

Bates, J.A.V., and P. W. Mathan. Transcutaneous electrical nerve stimulation for chronic pain. *Anaesthesia* 35 (1980): 817.

Bauer, Cathryn. *Acupressure for Everyone.* New York: Henry Holt, 1991.

Bean, Constance A. *The Better Back Book.* New York: William Morrow, 1989.

Benson, Herbert, M.D. *The Relaxation Response.* New York: Morrow & Co., 1975.

Borenstein, David, et al. *Low Back Pain: Medical Diagnosis and Comprehensive Management.* 2d ed., Philadelphia: W. B. Saunders, 1995.

Borysenko, Joan. *Minding the Body, Mending the Mind.* Toronto/New York: Bantam Books, 1988.

———. *The Power of the Mind to Heal.* Carson, CA: Hay House, 1994.

Burn, Loic. *A Manual of Medical Manipulation.* Dordrecht, The Netherlands: Kluwer Academic Publishers, 1994.

The Burton Goldberg Group. *Alternative Medicine: The Definitive Guide.* Puyallup, WA: Futura Medicine Publishing, 1994.

Bzdek, V., and E. Keller. Effects of therapeutic touch on tension headache pain. *Nursing Research* 35 (1986): 101–106.

Calliet, Rene, M.D. *Low Back Pain Syndrome.* 5th ed., Philadelphia: F. A. Davis, 1995.

Cherkin, Daniel C., and Frederick A. MacCormack. Patient evaluations of low back pain care from family physicians and chiropractors. *Western Journal of Medicine* 150 (1989): 351–55.

Chopra, Deepak, M.D. *Ageless Body, Timeless Mind.* New York: Harmony Books, 1993.

*Conn's Current Therapy.* Philadelphia: W. B. Saunders, 1994.

Cowles, Jane. *Pain Relief.* New York: MasterMedia Ltd., 1993.

DuBois, J. Robert. *Back Talk.* Port Henry, N.Y.: Bannister Publications, 1987.

Elias, Jason, and Shelagh Masline. *Healing Herbal Remedies.* New York: Dell, 1995.

Feltman, John, ed. *Hands-on Healing.* Emmaus, PA: Rodale Press, 1989.

Fezler, William. *Creative Imagery.* New York: Simon & Schuster, 1989.

Fields, Rick, et al., eds. *Chop Wood, Carry Water: A Guide to*

*Finding Spiritual Fulfillment in Everyday Life*. Los Angeles: J. P. Tarcher, 1986.

Findlay, S., et al. Wonder Cures from the Fringe. *US News & World Report* 3, no. 13 (23 September 1991): 68–74.

Fischer, A. A., and C. H. Chang. Electromyographic evidence of paraspinal muscle spasm during sleep in patients with low back pain. *Clin. J. Pain* 1 (1985): 147.

*The Fit Back*. Alexandria, VA: Time-Life Books, 1988.

Fox, E. J., and R. Melzack. Transcutaneous electrical nerve stimulation and acupuncture: Comparison of treatment for low back pain. *Pain* 2 (1976): 141–48.

Gach, Michael Reed. *Acupressure's Potent Points: A Guide to Self-Care for Common Ailments*. New York: Bantam, 1990.

———. *The Bum Back Book*. Berkeley, CA: Celestial Arts, 1983.

Gaines, MaryBeth Pappas. *Fantastic Water Workouts*. Champaign, IL: Human Kinetics, 1993.

Gianakopoulos, G., et al. Inversion devices: Their roles in producing lumbar distraction. *Arch. Phys. Med. Rehab.* 66: 100, 1985.

Gray, Timothy J. *Back Works*. Seattle: BookPartners, 1993.

Green, Lawrence E. *The Bad Back Diet Book*. San Francisco: Chronicle Books, 1987.

Guiness, Alma E., ed. *Family Guide to Natural Medicine*. Pleasantville, NY: Reader's Digest Association, 1993.

Haldeman, S., et al. *Guidelines for Chiropractic Quality Assurance and Practice Parameters*. Gaithersburg, MD: Aspen Publishers, 1992.

Heidt, P. Effect of therapeutic touch on anxiety level of hospitalized patients. *Nursing Research* 30 (1981): 32–37.

Hochschuler, Stephen, M.D. *A Back Owner's Manual*. Texas Back Institute. Boston: Houghton Mifflin, 1991.

Hooper, Paul D. *Preventing Low Back Pain*. Baltimore: Williams & Wilkins, 1992.

Hu, S. Positive thinking reduces heart rate and fear responses to speech-phobic imagery. *Perceptual & Motion Skills* (December 1992): 1067–73.

Hutson, M. A. *Back Pain: Recognition and Management*. Oxford: Butterworth Heinemann, 1993.

Imrie, David, and Lu Barbuto. *The Back Power Program*. New York: Wiley & Sons, 1990.

Jetter, Judy, and Nancy Kadlec. *Bathtub Exercises for Arthritis and Back Pain*. New York: Dutton, 1986.

Kastner, Mark. *Alternative Healing*. La Mesa, CA: Halcyon Publishing, 1993.

Khalil, Terek M., et al. *Ergonomics in Back Pain: A Guide to Prevention and Rehabilitation*. New York: Van Nostrand Reinhold, 1993.

Krieger, D. Therapeutic touch: The imprimatur of nursing. *Am. J. Nursing* 75 (1975): 784–87.

Krieger, D., E. Peper, and S. Ancoli. Therapeutic touch: Searching for evidence of physiological change. *Am. J. Nursing* 79 (1979): 660–62.

Krumhanal, Bernice, and Charles Nowacek. Case study—Spinal manipulation under anaesthesia. *Physical Therapy Forum*, vol. 4, September 1989.

Kuo, Simmone. *Long Life, Good Health Through Tai-Chi Chuan*. Berkeley, CA: North Atlantic Books, 1991.

Landon, B. R. Heat or cold for the relief of low back pain? *Phys. Ther.* 47 (1967): 1126.

Leibowitz, Judith, and Bill Connington. *The Alexander Technique*. New York: Harper & Row, 1990.

Lessell, Dr. Colin B. *The World Travellers' Manual of Homeopathy*. Essex, Eng.: C. W. Daniel Company, Ltd., 1993.

Lewith, George, M.D., and Sandra Horn. *Drug-Free Pain Relief: A Self-Help Guide*. Rochester, VT: Thorsons Publishers, 1987.

Lu, Henry C. *Chinese System of Food Cures: Prevention and Remedies*. New York: Sterling Publishing, 1986.

Macrae, Janet. *Therapeutic Touch: A Practical Guide*. New York: Knopf, 1988.

Marcus, Paul. *Thorson's Introduction Guide to Acupuncture*. London: HarperCollins, 1991.

Margolis, Simeon, and Hamilton Moses III. *The Johns Hopkins Medical Handbook*. New York: Medletter Associates, 1992.

Marti, James E. *Alternative Health & Medicine Encyclopedia*. Detroit: Visible Ink, 1995.

Mead, Mark. Chiropractic's New Haven. *East West,* November 1989.

Meade, T. W., et al. Low back pain of mechanical origin: Randomised comparison of chiropractic and hospital outpatient treatment. *British Medical Journal* 300 (1990): 1431–37.

Melzack, R., et al. Trigger points and acupuncture points for pain: Correlations and implications. *Pain* 3 (1977): 3–23.

———. Transcutaneous electrical nerve stimulation for low back pain. A comparison of TENS and massage for pain and range of motion. *Phys. Ther.* 6 (1983): 489–93.

Mills, Simon, and Steven J. Finando. *Alternatives in Healing.* New York: NAL Books, 1988.

Naparstek, Belleruth. *Staying Well with Guided Imagery.* New York: Time Warner, 1994.

Ody, Penelope. *The Complete Medicinal Herbal.* New York: Dorling Kindersley, 1993.

Oliver, Jean. *Back Care: An Illustrated Guide.* Oxford, Eng.: Butterworth-Heineman, 1994.

Pelletier, Kenneth R. *Mind as Healer, Mind as Slayer.* Rev. ed. New York: Delacorte, 1992.

Phillips, Robert H. *Coping with Rheumatoid Arthritis.* Garden City Park, NY: Avery, 1988.

Porter, Richard W. *Management of Back Pain.* Edinburgh, NY: Churchill Livingstone, 1993.

*Prevention* editors. *The Complete Book of Natural and Medicinal Cures.* Emmaus, PA: Rodale, 1994.

Prudden, Bonnie. *Myotherapy: Bonnie Prudden's Complete Guide to Pain-Free Living.* New York: Ballantine, 1980.

———. *Pain Erasure: The Bonnie Prudden Way.* New York: Ballantine, 1980.

Quinn J. Therapeutic touch as energy exchange: Testing the theory. *Advances in Nursing Science* 6 (1984): 42–49.

Roberts, D. J., et al. Relief of chronic low back pain: Heat versus cold. In Aronoff, G. M. (ed.), *Evaluation and Treatment of Chronic Pain,* pp. 263–66. Baltimore: Urban & Schwarzenberg, 1985.

Root, Leon, M.D. *No More Aching Back*. New York: Villard Books, 1990.

Rose, Dr. Barry. *The Family Health Guide to Homeopathy*. Berkeley, CA: Celestial Arts, 1992.

Sarno, John, M.D. *Mind Over Back Pain*. New York: William Morrow, 1984.

Schatz, Dr. Mary Pullig. *Back Care Basics*. Berkeley, CA: Rodmell Press, 1992.

Siegel, Bernie, M.D. *Love, Medicine & Miracles*. New York: Harper & Row, 1986.

Sjolund, B., et al. Increased cerebrospinal fluid levels of endorphins after electroacupuncture. *Acta. Physiol. Scand.* 100 (1977): 382–84.

Smith, Dr. Trevor. *Homeopathic Medicine*. Rochester, VT: Healing Arts Press, 1989.

Sobel, Dava, and Arthur Klein. *Backache: What Exercises Work*. New York: St. Martin's, 1994.

Spiegel, David, et al. Effect of psychosocial treatment on survival of patients with metastatic breast cancer. *Lancet* (1989): 888–91.

Stein, Diane. *All Women Are Healers*. Freedom, CA: Crossing Press, 1990.

Sutton, Nigel. *Applied Tai Chi Chuan*. London: A&C Black, 1991.

*Taber's Cyclopedic Medical Dictionary*, 16th ed. Philadelphia: F. A. Davis, 1989.

Tierra, Michael. *The Way of Herbs*. New York: Washington Square Press, 1983.

Trager, Milton. *Trager Mentastics: Movements as a Way to Agelessness*. Barrytown, NY: Station Hill Press, 1987.

Trattler, Dr. Ross. *Better Health Through Natural Healing*. New York: McGraw-Hill, 1985.

van der Wiel, H. E., et al. Biochemical parameters of bone turnover during ten days of bed rest and subsequent mobilization. *Bone Mineralization* 13 (1991): 123–29.

Walker, Morton, D.P.M. Nature's healer, DMSO. *Healthy & Natural Journal* 2 (1995): 58–62, 139.

Weil, Andrew, M.D. *Natural Health, Natural Medicine*. Boston: Houghton Mifflin, 1990.

Weiner, Michael, and Kathleen Goss. *The Complete Book of Homeopathy*. Garden City Park, NY: Avery, 1989.

White, Arthur H., and Jerome A. Schofferman, eds. *Spine Care: Diagnosis and Conservative Treatment*. vol. 1. St. Louis: Mosby-Year Book, 1995.

White, Arthur, and Robert Anderson, eds. *Conservative Care of Low Back Pain*. Baltimore: Williams & Wilkins, 1991.

White, Augustus A., M.D. *Your Aching Back: A Doctor's Guide to Relief*. New York: Simon & Schuster, 1990.

White, Martha. *Water Exercise*. Champaign, IL: Human Kinetics, 1995.

Wilen, Joan, and Lydia Wilen. *Live and Be Well*. New York: HarperCollins, 1992.

Winter, Ruth. *Consumer's Dictionary of Medicines*. New York: Crown, 1993.

Zimmerman, Julie. *The Almanac of Back Pain Treatments*. Brunswick, ME: Biddle Publishing, 1991.

———. *Chronic Back Pain: Moving On*. Brunswick, ME: Biddle Publishing, 1991.

———. *The Diagnosis and Misdiagnosis of Back Pain*. Brunswick, ME: Biddle Publishing, 1991.

## Additional Suggested Readings

Achterberg, Jeanne, Ph.D. *Rituals of Healing: Using Imagery for Health and Wellness*. New York: Bantam Books, 1994.

Alexander, F. M. *Constructive Conscious Control of the Individual*. Long Beach, CA: Centerline Press, 1985. First published in 1923 by E. P. Dutton.

———. *Use of the Self*. London: Victor Gollancz, 1985.

Alman, Brian M. *Self-Hypnosis: The Complete Manual*. New York: Brunner/Mazel, 1992.

Amhui Medical School Hospital, China, comp. *Chinese Massage: A Handbook of Therapeutic Massage*. Point Roberts, WA: Hartley & Marks, 1987.

Anderson, Robert A., M.D. *Wellness Medicine*. New Canaan, Conn.: Keat Publishing, 1990.

Aston Training Center. *Aston-Patterning*. Incline Village, NV, 1987.

Benson, Herbert, M.D. *The Wellness Book*. New York: Carol Publishing Group, 1992.

Byers, Dwight. *Better Health with Foot Reflexology*. Available through the International Institute of Reflexology, PO Box 12642, St. Petersburg, FL 33733-2642.

Caplan, Deborah. *Back Trouble: A New Approach to Prevention and Recovery Based on the Alexander Technique*. Gainesville, FL: Triad Publishing, 1987.

Carper, Jean. *Food—Your Miracle Medicine: How Food Can Prevent & Cure Over 100 Symptoms & Problems*. San Francisco: HarperCollins, 1993.

Chopra, Deepak, M.D. *Perfect Health: The Complete Mind/Body Guide*. New York: Harmony Books, 1991.

———. *Quantum Healing: Exploring the Frontiers of Body, Mind, Medicine*. New York: Bantam Books, 1993.

Clark, Barbara. *Jin Shin Acutouch: The Tai Chi of Healing Arts*. San Diego, CA: Clark Publishing, 1987.

Cohen, Sherry. *The Magic of Touch*. New York: Harper & Row, 1987.

Cousins, Norman. *Head First: The Biology of Hope and the Healing Power of the Human Spirit*. New York: Viking, 1990.

Edlin, Gordon, and Eric Golanty. *Health and Wellness: A Holistic Approach*. Boston, MA: Jones & Bartlett Publishers, 1992.

Fanning, Patrick. *Visualization for Change*. Oakland, CA: New Harbinger, 1988.

Feldenkrais, Moshe. *Easy to Do Exercises to Improve Posture, Vision, Imagination and Personal Awareness*. San Francisco: Harper, 1991.

Findlay, S., et al. Wonder Cures from the Fringe. *U.S. News & World Report* 3, no. 13 (23 September 1991): 68–74.

Goldstein, Joseph, and Jack Kornfield. *Seeking the Heart of Wisdom*. Boston: Shambhala, 1987.

Goleman, Daniel. *The Meditative Mind*. Los Angeles: J. P. Tarcher, 1988.

Goleman, Daniel, and Joel Gurin, eds. *Mind/Body Medicine.* Yonkers, NY: Consumers Reports Book, 1993.

Green, Elmer. *Beyond Biofeedback.* New York: Delacorte, 1977.

Grossinger, Richard. *Homeopathy: An Introduction for Skeptics and Beginners.* Berkeley, CA: North Atlantic Books, 1993.

Hahnemann, Samuel. *Organon of Medicine.* Translated by W. Boericke, M.D. New Delhi: B. Jain Publishers, 1992.

Heimlich, Jane. *What Your Doctor Won't Tell You.* New York: Harper Perennial, 1990.

Hoffman, David. *The New Holistic Herbal.* Rockport, MA: Element Books, 1992.

Horay, Patrick, and David Harp. *Hot Water Therapy.* Oakland, CA: New Harbinger, 1991.

Kabat-Zinn, Jon. *Full Catastrophic Living: Using the Wisdom of Your Body and Mind to Face Stress, Pain, and Illness.* New York: Delacorte Press, 1990.

Kaptchuk, Ted. *The Web That Has No Weaver: Understanding Chinese Medicine.* New York: Congdon & Weed, 1993.

Kittredge, Mary. *Pain.* New York: Chelsea House Publishers, 1992.

Klaper, Michael, M.D. *Vegan Nutrition Pure and Simple.* Maui, HI: Gentle World, 1987.

Krieger, Dolores. *The Therapeutic Touch: How to Use Your Hands to Help or to Heal.* Englewood Cliffs, N.J.: Prentice-Hall, 1979.

Kunz, Kevin, and Barbara Kunz. *Hand and Foot Reflexology: A Self-Help Guide.* Englewood Cliffs, NJ: Prentice-Hall, 1984.

Kushi, Michio. *The Macrobiotic Way: The Complete Macrobiotic Diet and Exercise Book.* Wayne, NJ: Avery Publishing, 1985.

McDonald, Kathleen. *How to Meditate.* Boston: Wisdom Publications, 1992.

Manheim, Carol J., et al. *Craniosacral Therapy and SomatoEmotional Release: The Self-Healing Body.* Thorofare, NJ: SLACK Inc., 1989.

Melzack, R., and P. D. Wall. Pain mechanisms: A new theory. *Science* 150 (1965).

Michalak, Patricia. *Rodale's Successful Organic Gardening: Herbs.* Emmaus, PA: Rodale Press, 1993.

Mindell, Earl, R.Ph., Ph.D. *Earl Mindell's Herb Bible*. New York: Simon & Schuster, 1992.

Monte, Tom, et al. *World Medicine: The East West Guide to Healing Your Body*. New York: Jeremy Tarcher, 1993.

Moore, Michael. *Medicinal Plants of the Desert and Canyon West*. Santa Fe, NM: Museum of New Mexico Press, 1989.

Murray, Michael. *Natural Alternatives to Over-the-Counter and Prescription Drugs*. New York: William Morrow, 1994.

Murray, Michael, and Joseph Pizzorno. *Encyclopedia of Natural Medicine*. Rocklin, CA: Prima Publishing, 1991.

National Center for Homeopathy. *Homeopathy: Natural Medicine for the 21st Century*. Alexandria, VA, 1990.

Panos, Maesimund B., and Jane Heimlich. *Homeopathic Medicine at Home*. Los Angeles: J. P. Tarcher, 1980.

Reid, Daniel. *Chinese Herbal Medicine*. Boston: Shambhala Publications, 1993.

Robbins, John. *May All Be Fed*. New York: Morrow, 1992; Avon, 1993.

Rossman, Martin L., M.D. *Healing Yourself: A Step-by-Step Program for Better Health Through Imagery*. New York: Walker & Co., 1987.

Schein, Jeffrey, and Philip Hansten. *Consumer's Guide to Drug Interactions*. New York: Collier Books, 1993.

Sherman, John A., N.D. *The Complete Botanical Prescriber*. Compiled by John A. Sherman, 1993.

Sivananda Yoga Vedanta Center. *Learn Yoga in a Weekend*. New York: Knopf, 1993.

Tappan, Frances M. *Healing Massage Techniques*. Appleton & Lange, 1988.

Teschler, Wilfried. *The Polarity Healing Handbook*. San Leandro, CA: Interbook, Inc., 1986.

Tierra, Lesley. *The Herbs of Life: Health and Healing Using Western and Chinese Techniques*. Freedom, CA: The Crossing Press, 1992.

Tyler, Varro E. *The Honest Herbal*, 3rd ed. Binghamton, NY: Haworth Press, 1993.

Ulman, Dana. *Discovering Homeopathy*. Berkeley, CA: North Atlantic Books, 1991.

Upledger Institute. *Discover the CranioSacral System.* Palm Beach Gardens, FL, 1991.

Weil, Andrew, M.D. *Spontaneous Healing.* Boston: Houghton Mifflin, 1994.

Weinman, Ric A. *Your Hands Can Heal: Learn to Channel Healing Energy.* New York: E. P. Dutton, 1988.

# INDEX

# ABOUT THE AUTHOR

**Deborah Mitchell** is a writer and editor whose medical and health-related articles have appeared in several consumer and professional journals, including *Internal Medicine World Report, Geriatrics, Hospital Formulary, Geriatrics Medicine News & Reports,* and *Organic Digest.* She has ghostwritten or coauthored five books, including *The Good Sex Book: Recovering and Discovering Your Sexual Self* and *The Natural Health Guide to Headache Relief.* Deborah lives and works in Tucson, Arizona.